Motivational Interviewing with Teens Made Simple

A Step-by-Step Training Guide for Parents, Counselors, and Youth Workers

I0039084

Honor Victoria Frost

ISBN: 978-1-7642720-8-7

Table of Contents

Preface

The conversation happens every day in homes, schools, and youth programs across the country. An adult notices a teenager making choices that seem self-destructive or counterproductive. The adult, motivated by genuine care and concern, launches into an explanation of why the teenager should change their behavior. The teenager responds with silence, arguments, or outright defiance. The adult tries harder, speaking louder or imposing consequences. The teenager withdraws further. Both parties walk away frustrated, and nothing changes.

This pattern isn't the result of bad intentions or inadequate caring. It stems from a fundamental misunderstanding about how change actually happens, particularly during adolescence. Most adults approach teenagers with strategies that worked when those teens were children, not recognizing that the adolescent brain operates under different rules entirely.

Motivational Interviewing offers a different approach. Developed by psychologists William Miller and Stephen Rollnick, MI recognizes that lasting change comes from within individuals, not from external pressure. This approach has been extensively researched and proven effective across multiple populations and settings. Yet despite its success with adolescents in clinical trials, MI techniques remain largely unknown to the parents, counselors, and youth workers who interact with teenagers daily.

This book bridges that gap. It translates evidence-based motivational interviewing principles into practical strategies that busy adults can learn and implement immediately. The techniques presented here don't require advanced training or perfect execution. They require only a willingness to approach teenagers differently – with curiosity rather than judgment, collaboration rather than control, and patience for the developmental process that is adolescence.

The title includes "Made Simple" because complexity often prevents implementation. Many excellent books about motivational interviewing exist, but most assume clinical training and therapeutic settings. Real-world interactions with teenagers happen in kitchens and classrooms, in cars and community centers. They happen when adults are tired, frustrated, or pressed for time. The approaches in this book are designed for these real conditions.

This is not a book about permissive parenting or abandoning adult responsibility. MI maintains clear boundaries and expectations while changing how we communicate about them. The goal isn't to eliminate all conflict with teenagers – some conflict is developmentally normal and even beneficial. The goal is to have conflicts that lead somewhere productive rather than just creating more distance and resistance.

The case examples throughout this book represent composites drawn from years of working with families, schools, and youth organizations. Names and identifying details have been changed to protect privacy, but the interactions reflect common patterns that most adults who work with teenagers will recognize.

This book is written for three primary audiences, each bringing different strengths to their work with adolescents. Parents possess the advantage of long-term relationships and deep emotional investment. Professional counselors bring training in human development and therapeutic communication. Youth workers contribute expertise in group dynamics and program implementation. All three groups share the common challenge of connecting with teenagers in ways that support growth while respecting developing autonomy.

The techniques presented here work because they align with how teenagers actually think and communicate, rather than how adults wish they would. They account for the neurobiological realities of adolescent development, the social pressures that define teenage experience, and the identity formation processes that make this stage of life both challenging and full of potential.

Change is always possible, but it rarely happens through argument or coercion. It happens through connection, understanding, and the careful cultivation of internal motivation. The strategies in this book provide pathways to those connections, even with the most resistant teenagers.

The investment required is primarily one of perspective rather than time. Learning to ask different questions, listen more carefully, and respond with curiosity rather than immediate solutions doesn't take longer than traditional approaches. Often, it takes less time because it leads to more productive conversations and fewer repeated conflicts.

Most importantly, these techniques work not because they manipulate teenagers into compliance, but because they honor the developmental process of becoming an independent adult. They recognize that the ultimate goal isn't obedience, but rather the development of internal motivation, decision-making skills, and the capacity for authentic relationships that will serve young people throughout their lives.

The pages that follow provide concrete tools for achieving these outcomes. They offer hope for adults who have felt stuck in unproductive patterns with the teenagers they care about. Most significantly, they provide a foundation for relationships that can weather the storms of adolescence and emerge stronger on the other side.

Section 1: Part I: Understanding Teen Resistance

Chapter 1: The Teenage Brain on Ambivalence

Picture Sarah, a 16-year-old who desperately wants to improve her grades but can't seem to put down her phone long enough to study. One moment she's motivated to change, creating elaborate study schedules and downloading productivity apps. The next moment, she's scrolling through TikTok at 2 AM, knowing she has a test tomorrow. Her parents are baffled. Her teachers are frustrated. And Sarah? She's caught in a whirlwind of wanting to change while simultaneously resisting it.

This isn't defiance or laziness – it's **ambivalence**, and it's hardwired into the teenage brain. Understanding why teens feel torn between change and staying the same isn't just helpful; it's essential for anyone working with adolescents.

The Architecture of the Adolescent Mind

The teenage brain is essentially under construction, with major renovations happening in the most important areas. While adults often view teen behavior as irrational or inconsistent, neuroscience reveals that adolescents are operating with brains that are literally still being built.

The **prefrontal cortex** – the brain's CEO responsible for executive functions, impulse control, and long-term planning – doesn't fully mature until around age 25 (Steinberg, 2013). Meanwhile, the **limbic system**, which processes emotions and drives reward-seeking behavior, is in overdrive during adolescence. This creates what researchers call the "maturational imbalance," where teens feel emotions intensely but lack the cognitive tools to regulate them effectively.

Think of it like having a Ferrari engine with bicycle brakes. The emotional accelerator is fully functional, but the rational braking system is still being installed. This biological reality explains why your teenager can passionately commit to a goal on Monday and completely abandon it by Wednesday – not because they don't care, but because their brain is literally changing how they process decisions from day to day.

Decision-Making in the Developing Brain

Adolescent decision-making operates on a fundamentally different system than adult cognition. Research by Laurence Steinberg and his colleagues has identified several key differences that directly impact how teens approach change:

The Reward Sensitivity Peak: During adolescence, the brain's reward system becomes hyperactive. Dopamine receptors in areas associated with pleasure and motivation multiply rapidly, making teens more sensitive to potential rewards than either children or adults (Steinberg et al., 2018). This means the immediate gratification of staying in their comfort zone often outweighs the distant benefits of change.

Social Brain Activation: The teenage brain shows heightened activity in regions associated with social cognition when peers are present or even just imagined (Blakemore, 2018). A teen might genuinely want to change their study habits, but when friends text about a party, their brain literally prioritizes social connection over academic goals.

Hot vs. Cool Processing: Adolescents have two distinct decision-making modes. "Cool" cognition happens in calm, supportive environments and resembles adult-like rational thinking. "Hot" cognition kicks in during emotional or social situations, leading to more impulsive choices. The problem? Most real-world decisions happen in "hot" contexts (Casey et al., 2019).

Consider Marcus, a 17-year-old who desperately wants to quit vaping. In his room at night, planning his quit strategy, his "cool" brain creates detailed plans and feels confident about change. But when he's stressed at school and his friends offer him a vape, his "hot" brain takes over, prioritizing immdiate relief and social acceptance over his long-term goals.

The Neurobiology of Ambivalence

Ambivalence isn't a character flaw – it's a neurobiological reality. The teenage brain is simultaneously driven by multiple, often competing systems:

The Approach System: Located primarily in the ventral striatum, this system drives teens toward rewarding experiences and novel situations. It whispers, "Go for it! Try something new! Take that risk!"

The Avoidance System: Centered in the amygdala and related structures, this system warns against potential threats and negative outcomes. It shouts, "Wait! This could go wrong! Stay safe!"

The Cognitive Control System: Based in the prefrontal cortex, this system tries to weigh options rationally and make planned decisions. But remember – it's still under construction.

When teens experience ambivalence about change, these systems are literally battling in their brains. The approach system might be excited about the benefits of change, while the avoidance system fears the unknown consequences. Meanwhile, the cognitive control system is trying to referee a fight it's not quite equipped to handle.

This explains why conversations about change with teens can feel like emotional whiplash. They're not being manipulative or indecisive – their brains are genuinely experiencing conflicting neural signals about the same situation.

Identity Formation and Change Resistance

Adolescence is the critical period for identity development, and this process profoundly affects how teens approach change. Erik Erikson's concept of "identity vs. role confusion" takes on new meaning when viewed through the lens of brain development (Erikson, 1968).

The Identity Paradox: Teens simultaneously need to figure out who they are while being asked to change who they are. This creates an inherent tension. When adults suggest changes, teens may interpret this as criticism of their emerging identity rather than helpful guidance.

Stability Seeking: While teens appear to crave novelty, they also desperately need some sense of stability during this turbulent period. Current behaviors and patterns, even problematic ones, provide a familiar foundation in a world where everything else feels uncertain. Asking teens to change can feel like asking them to abandon one of the few consistent things in their lives.

Autonomy Development: The drive toward independence is neurologically programmed during adolescence. When change suggestions come from adults, teens' brains may automatically trigger resistance simply because the ideas originated externally. This isn't about the merit of the change itself – it's about protecting their developing sense of autonomy.

Take Emma, a 15-year-old whose grades are slipping because she stays up late texting friends. Her parents want her to change her sleep schedule, but Emma experiences this as an attack on her social connections – a core part of her identity. The suggestion to go to bed earlier isn't just about sleep; it threatens her sense of who she is as someone who's always available for her friends.

The Social Context of Teen Change

Unlike adults, teenagers don't make change decisions in isolation. The adolescent brain is exquisitely attuned to social information, making peer relationships a critical factor in any change process.

Social Threat Detection: Research shows that social rejection activates the same brain regions as physical pain in teenagers (Gunther Moor et al., 2012). This means that changes which might affect peer relationships are processed as literal threats to survival. A teen considering changing their friend group to support healthier choices faces genuine neurological distress.

Identity Mirroring: Teens use peer relationships as mirrors to understand themselves. When they consider changing, they're not just evaluating the change itself – they're wondering how it will affect how others see them and, by extension, how they see themselves.

Risk Assessment: The teenage brain calculates social risks differently than other types of risks. While an adult might worry about long-term health consequences of risky behavior, a teen's brain prioritizes the immediate social consequences of *not* engaging in that behavior.

Understanding Developmental Timing

Not all resistance to change is created equal. The timing of when change is introduced matters tremendously for adolescent brains.

Early Adolescence (11-14): The brain is beginning major reconstruction. Teens at this stage often experience dramatic mood swings and may seem to change their minds frequently. Ambivalence about change is intense because emotional systems are becoming more reactive while cognitive control systems are just beginning their renovation.

Middle Adolescence (15-17): Peak risk-taking period due to the maturational imbalance between emotional and cognitive systems. Teens may be most resistant to adult-initiated change during this period because their drive for autonomy is strongest while their capacity for long-term thinking is still limited.

Late Adolescence (18-21): Cognitive control systems are becoming more mature, making this an optimal time for supporting lasting change. Teens can better integrate emotional and rational information, though peer influence remains significant.

Understanding these developmental windows helps explain why the same teen might be receptive to change conversations at one age but completely resistant just months later. It's not personal – it's neurological.

The Default Mode Network

Recent neuroscience research has identified the "default mode network" – a set of brain regions active when we're not focused on specific tasks. In adolescents, this network shows unique patterns that affect how they approach change.

The teenage default mode network is hyperactive in areas associated with social cognition and self-referential thinking (Blakemore & Mills, 2014). This means that when teens aren't actively engaged in tasks, their brains automatically shift to thinking about social relationships and how they fit into their peer groups.

This has profound implications for change conversations. When teens seem distracted or resistant during discussions about change, their brains may literally be defaulting to social concerns. They're not ignoring the conversation – they're processing it through a neural filter that prioritizes social implications above all else.

Practical Implications for Adults

Understanding the neuroscience of teen ambivalence doesn't excuse problematic behavior, but it does inform how we approach change conversations. Here are key insights for working with adolescent brains:

Expect Inconsistency: Teen commitment to change will naturally fluctuate based on their emotional state, social context, and even time of day. This isn't a sign of failure – it's normal brain development.

Time It Right: Approach change conversations when teens are in "cool" emotional states, not during times of stress or social activation. This might mean waiting until after the friend drama settles or choosing moments when they're not rushing to school.

Address Social Concerns: Always explore how potential changes might affect peer relationships. If you don't help teens problem-solve the social implications of change, their brains will default to protecting social connections over implementing new behaviors.

Validate Ambivalence: Instead of pushing through ambivalence, acknowledge it as normal and expected. "It makes sense that part of you wants to change and part of you doesn't – that's how most people feel about change."

Support Identity Integration: Help teens see how change aligns with their values and emerging identity rather than threatening it. "How does improving your grades fit with your goal of becoming a veterinarian?"

Moving Forward with Brain-Based Understanding

The teenage brain's relationship with change is complex, but it's not hopeless. By understanding the neurobiological underpinnings of adolescent ambivalence, we can approach teens with compassion rather than frustration.

Remember that every time a teen experiences ambivalence about change, their brain is doing exactly what it's supposed to do developmentally. They're weighing immediate versus long-term rewards, considering social implications, protecting their emerging identity, and trying to integrate competing neural signals – all with a prefrontal cortex that's still under construction.

This understanding transforms how we view teen "resistance." Instead of seeing defiance or laziness, we can recognize a developing brain trying to navigate complex decisions with limited cognitive resources. This shift in perspective opens up new possibilities for connection and support.

Whether you're a parent, counselor, or teacher, approaching teen ambivalence with neurobiological understanding changes everything. You're not fighting against a stubborn teenager – you're supporting a developing brain through one of the most challenging periods of human development. That requires patience, compassion, and strategies specifically designed for adolescent neurobiology.

The next step is learning how to communicate with these developing brains in their native language – and that means understanding how digital natives process and share information.

Chapter 2: Digital Native Communication

Seventeen-year-old Jake can maintain simultaneous conversations with eight different friends across four different platforms while watching Netflix and completing homework. His mother struggles to get his attention for a five-minute face-to-face conversation. When she finally sits him down to talk about his grades, Jake's responses are monosyllabic and he seems completely disengaged. She wonders if he even cares about his future.

Here's what's really happening: Jake's brain has been shaped by digital communication from early childhood. He processes information differently, builds relationships through screens, and expresses emotions through memes and emojis. When his mother tries to have a traditional heart-to-heart conversation, she's essentially speaking a foreign language to his neurologically adapted brain.

This isn't about teenagers being addicted to technology or losing social skills. Today's adolescents are the first generation of true digital natives – their brains have developed alongside smartphones, social media, and instant connectivity. Understanding how to meet them in their communication style isn't about giving up on face-to-face interaction; it's about building bridges that lead to meaningful connection.

The Digital Native Brain

Digital natives don't just use technology differently – they think differently. Research by Gary Small and colleagues at UCLA found that internet searching actually changes brain activity patterns, particularly in areas responsible for decision-making and complex reasoning (Small et al., 2009). Teens who grew up with smartphones show enhanced activity in regions associated with visual processing and task-switching, but decreased activity in areas linked to deep reading and sustained attention.

Parallel Processing: Unlike previous generations who learned to focus on one task at a time, digital natives have developed enhanced ability to manage multiple information streams simultaneously. Their brains have adapted to process fragmented information quickly rather than engaging in sustained, linear thinking.

Visual Communication: Teens communicate increasingly through images, videos, and visual symbols. A single meme can convey complex emotional states that might take paragraphs to explain in traditional conversation. Their brains have become highly skilled at encoding and decoding visual information rapidly.

Asynchronous Relationship Building: Digital natives build relationships through ongoing, asynchronous communication rather than scheduled, focused interactions. They maintain emotional intimacy through constant, brief touchpoints rather than lengthy conversations.

Context Switching: Teenage brains have become exceptionally good at rapidly switching between different communication contexts – adjusting tone, content, and presentation style based on platform and audience almost instantaneously.

Understanding Teen Communication Styles

To communicate effectively with digital natives, we need to understand how their communication patterns differ from traditional models:

Brevity as Intimacy: Short messages aren't signs of disinterest – they're efficiency. Teens can convey deep emotional connection through carefully chosen words, emojis, or even the timing of their responses. A "k" might seem dismissive to adults, but in teen communication, it can signal understanding, agreement, or even affection depending on context.

Emoji Emotional Language: For digital natives, emojis aren't decorations – they're emotional punctuation. The difference between "good job" and "good job 😊" represents entirely different emotional messages. Teens often feel that text without emojis lacks emotional warmth or seems overly formal.

Layered Communication: Digital natives rarely communicate on just one level. They might be responding to your text while simultaneously commenting on a friend's social media post and listening to music. This isn't distraction – it's their normal state of multi-layered engagement.

Story-Based Sharing: Platforms like Instagram Stories and Snapchat have shaped how teens share experiences. They think in terms of moments, highlights, and visual narratives rather than chronological reporting. When adults ask "How was your day?" teens might struggle because their brains organize experiences as disconnected moments rather than linear stories.

Consider Maya, a 16-year-old whose parents worry she's not opening up about her anxiety. Maya posts vulnerable content on her private Instagram story regularly and has deep text conversations with friends about her mental health. When her parents try to have dinner table conversations about feelings, Maya shuts down – not because she's secretive, but because verbal, face-to-face emotional processing feels unnatural to her digitally-adapted communication style.

Platform-Specific Communication Patterns

Different digital platforms shape different aspects of teen communication. Understanding these patterns helps adults meet teens where they naturally express themselves:

Text Messaging: The most intimate digital space for teens. Text conversations often carry emotional weight similar to face-to-face conversations for previous generations. Response time, message length, and emoji choices all carry social and emotional significance.

Instagram: Curated self-presentation mixed with authentic moments through stories. Teens use Instagram to craft their ideal identity while also sharing genuine experiences with close friends through private stories and direct messages.

Snapchat: Immediate, ephemeral communication that feels safer for vulnerable sharing because messages disappear. Many teens prefer Snapchat for sensitive conversations because the temporary nature feels less risky than permanent text messages.

TikTok: Creative expression and community finding. Teens often discover identity and belonging through TikTok communities organized around shared interests, experiences, or identities. They may express aspects of themselves on TikTok that they don't share in person.

Discord: Deep community building around shared interests. For many teens, Discord servers provide more meaningful friendship connections than school-based relationships.

Understanding these platforms helps adults recognize where teens are having their most authentic conversations and emotional experiences. The key insight: teens aren't avoiding real communication by using these platforms – these platforms *are* their real communication.

Adapting Motivational Interviewing for Digital Communication

Traditional Motivational Interviewing relies heavily on verbal cues, nonverbal communication, and sustained conversation. Digital natives often struggle with these formats, but MI principles can be adapted for their communication preferences:

Micro-Conversations: Instead of expecting long, continuous discussions about change, break conversations into brief, focused exchanges spread over time. Send thoughtful questions via text and allow teens time to process and respond authentically.

Traditional MI: "Let's sit down and talk about your goals for this semester."

Digital-Adapted MI: "Been thinking about what you said yesterday about wanting to do better in math. What would 'better' look like to you?" (sent as text, allowing time for reflection)

Visual Processing: Use images, screenshots, or visual aids to help teens process complex emotions or decisions. Create simple charts or use drawing apps to explore ambivalence visually rather than only verbally.

Asynchronous Reflection: Digital natives often process emotions better when they have time to think and respond thoughtfully. Use voice messages, texts, or even shared documents to allow deeper reflection than real-time conversation permits.

Platform Matching: Meet teens on their preferred platforms for different types of conversations. They might prefer texting for emotional check-ins, FaceTime for problem-solving, or even using collaborative apps for goal-setting.

Building Rapport Through Digital Channels

Rapport with digital natives often builds differently than with previous generations. Understanding their relationship patterns helps adults connect more authentically:

Consistency Over Intensity: Digital natives build trust through regular, brief interactions rather than occasional deep conversations. Send consistent, supportive messages rather than waiting for major conversations.

Authenticity in Informality: Teens often interpret formal communication as distant or disconnected. Using their communication style (appropriate emojis, casual language, current references) signals respect for their cultural norms.

Responsive Availability: Digital natives expect responses within reasonable timeframes. While you don't need to be constantly available, acknowledging messages promptly helps build trust. Even a "got your message, let's talk more later" shows respect for their communication patterns.

Visual Engagement: Share images, memes, or visual content that connects to their interests. This shows you understand and value their visual communication style.

Cross-Platform Presence: Teens often feel more comfortable with adults who understand multiple platforms. You don't need to be active on every platform, but basic familiarity helps bridge generational communication gaps.

Navigating Digital Communication Challenges

Working with digital natives presents unique challenges that require adapted strategies:

Shortened Attention Spans: Digital natives have enhanced ability to process information quickly but may struggle with sustained attention. Keep key points concise and use multiple touchpoints rather than lengthy single conversations.

Solution: Break important conversations into segments. "We have three things to talk about. Let's start with the most important one and save the others for later."

Context Collapse: On digital platforms, different social contexts (family, friends, school) often collide, creating anxiety about authentic self-expression. Teens may struggle to communicate genuinely when they're worried about different audiences.

Solution: Create clearly defined communication spaces. "This conversation is just between us" or "I'm asking as your counselor, not sharing with parents."

Immediate Emotional Reactions: Digital communication can amplify emotional responses because teens can send messages immediately without cooling-off periods. This can escalate conflicts quickly.

Solution: Teach and model thoughtful response timing. "I can see you're upset. Take some time to think about what you want to say, and we can continue this conversation when you're ready."

Misreading Tone: Without facial expressions and voice tone, digital communication can lead to misunderstandings. Teens may interpret neutral messages as critical or dismissive.

Solution: Over-communicate positive intent. Use emoji, explicit positive language, and check for understanding. "I'm asking because I care about you, not because I'm judging."

Creating Digital Communication Agreements

Successful communication with digital natives often benefits from explicit agreements about how you'll interact:

Response Time Expectations: Clarify mutual expectations about response times. "I'll try to respond to texts within a few hours during weekdays, but weekend response might be slower."

Platform Preferences: Understand and respect teens' platform preferences for different types of conversations. "Would you prefer to text about this or talk in person?"

Privacy Boundaries: Clearly establish what communications will remain private and what might be shared with parents or other adults. "Our conversations stay between us unless you're in danger or ask me to share something."

Emergency Protocols: Establish clear guidelines for urgent situations. "If you need immediate help, call or text this number. For regular support, texting works great."

The Power of Memes and Metaphors

Digital natives often communicate complex emotions and concepts through memes, metaphors, and cultural references. Learning to speak this language opens doors to deeper connection:

Meme Literacy: Understanding popular memes helps adults connect with teen experiences. A teen sharing a "this is fine" meme while sitting in a burning room communicates overwhelming stress more effectively than saying "I'm stressed."

Cultural References: Staying aware of teen cultural touchstones (music, shows, online personalities) provides common ground for conversation and shows respect for their world.

Visual Metaphors: Use images, diagrams, or visual metaphors to explain complex concepts. Create simple infographics about change processes or use drawing apps to explore emotions visually.

Gaming Language: Many teens use gaming terminology to describe life experiences. Understanding concepts like "leveling up," "boss battles," and "side quests" helps adults speak their metaphorical language.

Balancing Digital and Face-to-Face Communication

The goal isn't to replace face-to-face communication but to use digital communication as a bridge to deeper connection:

Digital Warm-Up: Start conversations through teens' preferred digital channels before transitioning to in-person discussions. This allows them to process initially and come to face-to-face conversations more prepared.

Hybrid Conversations: Combine digital and in-person elements. Share articles, videos, or images via text, then discuss them in person. This gives teens preparation time while still prioritizing direct interaction.

Digital Documentation: Help teens document their growth and goals using digital tools they're comfortable with. Create shared documents, photo journals, or progress tracking apps that align with their technological comfort.

Screen-Free Agreements: Create specific times and spaces for device-free interaction, but frame these as special connection time rather than punishment or restriction.

Moving Into Identity-Focused Work

Understanding digital native communication is crucial, but it's only the foundation. Once adults can connect with teens through their preferred communication channels, the real work begins: helping them navigate the complex relationship between change and identity formation.

Digital natives face unique identity challenges because their self-exploration happens partly in public, permanent digital spaces. Their relationship with change is complicated by the fact that their identity experimentation is often documented, searchable, and socially visible in ways previous generations never experienced.

What This Means for Practice

Learning to communicate with digital natives isn't about becoming teenagers yourself or abandoning your professional boundaries. It's about recognizing that effective communication requires speaking in ways that align with how their brains have developed to process information.

When you text a thoughtful question instead of demanding immediate verbal response, when you acknowledge their emoji-rich messages as legitimate emotional communication, when you meet them on platforms where they feel comfortable expressing themselves – you're not enabling technology dependence. You're demonstrating respect for their neurological reality and creating conditions where meaningful change conversations can actually occur.

Chapter 3: Identity vs. Change

Sixteen-year-old Alex has been the "class clown" since middle school. Teachers know him as the kid who always has a joke ready, and friends count on him to lighten tense moments. But Alex is tired of being seen as unserious. He wants teachers to recognize his intelligence and peers to respect his opinions on important topics. When his school counselor suggests he try participating more genuinely in class discussions, Alex freezes up.

"But that's not who I am," he says. "Everyone expects me to be funny. If I start acting all serious and smart, people will think I'm fake or trying too hard."

Alex has hit the core dilemma of adolescent change: **How do you become who you want to be while maintaining who you've been?** This isn't simple teenage stubbornness – it's one of the most complex psychological challenges of human development. For teenagers, change isn't just about behavior modification; it's about identity reconstruction, and that process is both thrilling and terrifying.

The Adolescent Identity Construction Project

Erik Erikson identified adolescence as the critical period for resolving "identity vs. role confusion," but modern neuroscience reveals just how complex this process actually is (Erikson, 1968). The teenage brain is simultaneously trying to answer fundamental questions: *Who am I? Who do I want to become? How do others see me? Which version of myself is the "real" one?*

Identity as Ongoing Construction: Unlike children, who see identity as fairly fixed, or adults, who have established identity frameworks, teenagers experience identity as fluid and constantly evolving. This creates both opportunity and anxiety. They can experiment with different versions of themselves, but they also lack the stability of knowing who they "really" are.

Multiple Self-Concept Integration: Research by Susan Harter shows that adolescents develop multiple, sometimes contradictory self-concepts that they struggle to integrate (Harter, 2012). Alex might see himself as funny-with-friends, serious-with-family, creative-in-art-class, and anxious-about-college. Each context brings out different aspects of his personality, creating confusion about his "authentic" self.

Future Self Development: Teenagers are developing their capacity to imagine future versions of themselves, but this ability is still emerging. They can envision who they want to become but struggle to see concrete paths from their current identity to their desired identity.

This developmental reality means that when adults suggest changes to teenagers, they're not just asking them to modify behaviors – they're asking them to reconstruct their fundamental sense of self. No wonder teens resist.

How Identity Formation Complicates Change

The relationship between identity development and willingness to change creates several predictable challenges:

The Authenticity Trap: Teens often believe that "authentic" means staying consistent with who they've been. They may resist positive changes because these changes feel "fake" or like they're betraying their "true" selves. This is why Alex struggles with being more serious in class – it feels like pretending to be someone he's not.

Social Identity Pressure: During adolescence, peer relationships become central to identity development. Teens may resist changes that could affect how their friends see them, even when they genuinely want to change. The fear of social rejection often outweighs the desire for personal growth.

Identity Foreclosure vs. Identity Exploration: Some teens resolve identity anxiety by committing to a particular version of themselves too early (identity foreclosure), while others struggle with endless exploration without commitment (identity moratorium). Both states complicate change processes.

The Observer Effect: Teenagers are hyperaware that others are watching and evaluating their behavior. This "imaginary audience" phenomenon means they may avoid trying new behaviors because they're afraid of being seen as inconsistent or inauthentic.

Consider Maria, a 17-year-old who has always been the "responsible daughter" in her family. She manages her younger siblings, maintains perfect grades, and never causes problems. But Maria is burning out and wants to set boundaries, maybe even take some healthy risks like trying theater or dating. When her therapist explores these desires, Maria becomes anxious: "If I'm not the responsible one, who am I? My family needs me to be this way. And what if I try new things and I'm terrible at them? What if people see that I'm not as mature as they think?"

Maria's resistance to change isn't about laziness or fear of effort – it's about identity preservation. She's built her sense of self around being responsible and reliable. Changing these behaviors feels like losing herself entirely.

The Neurobiology of Identity and Change

Brain imaging studies reveal why identity concerns are so intense during adolescence and how they interact with change processes:

Heightened Self-Referential Processing: The adolescent brain shows increased activity in regions associated with self-referential thinking, particularly the medial prefrontal cortex (Blakemore & Mills, 2014). This means teens literally think about themselves more than children or adults do – not out of vanity, but because their brains are actively engaged in identity construction work.

Social Brain Sensitivity: Areas of the brain associated with social cognition and social evaluation (including the temporoparietal junction and superior temporal sulcus) are hyperactive during adolescence. This neurological reality means teens are constantly processing how others perceive them and how their behavior affects their social identity.

Reward System Identity Integration: The adolescent reward system doesn't just respond to external rewards – it's particularly sensitive to identity-consistent rewards. Behaviors that align with a teen's sense of self activate reward circuits more strongly than identity-inconsistent behaviors, even when the latter might lead to better outcomes.

Memory Consolidation of Identity Events: The adolescent brain prioritizes encoding and consolidating memories related to identity and social experiences. This means identity-relevant events (both positive and negative) have outsized impact on how teens see themselves and their capacity for change.

Working With Identity Development Rather Than Against It

Effective change work with teenagers requires understanding and respecting identity development processes rather than trying to override them:

Identity Integration vs. Identity Replacement: Instead of asking teens to abandon aspects of themselves, help them explore how desired changes can expand or integrate with existing identity elements. Alex doesn't need to stop being funny – he can explore being funny *and* intelligent, humorous *and* thoughtful.

Future Self Exploration: Help teens develop clearer, more detailed visions of their future selves that feel connected to their current identity. Use visualization exercises, letter-writing to future selves, or exploration of role models who embody both current and desired qualities.

Identity Flexibility Training: Teach teens that identity can be both stable and evolving. Help them understand that growth doesn't mean abandoning their core self – it means expanding their repertoire of ways to express that self.

Values-Based Change: Connect desired changes to teens' core values rather than external expectations. When changes align with their deepest values, they feel identity-consistent rather than identity-threatening.

Practical Strategies for Identity-Conscious Change Work

The Identity Integration Interview

When teens resist change because it feels inauthentic, try this structured exploration:

1. **Current Identity Appreciation**: "Tell me about the parts of yourself that you value most. What aspects of who you are do you never want to lose?"

2. **Future Self Visioning**: "When you imagine yourself five years from now, living the life you really want, what aspects of your current self are still there? What new aspects have developed?"

3. **Bridge Building**: "How might the changes we've been discussing help you become more fully yourself rather than less?"

4. **Integration Planning**: "What would it look like to make these changes in a way that honors who you are now while growing into who you want to become?"

The Authenticity Reframe

When teens worry that change means being "fake":

- **Expand the Definition**: "What if being authentic doesn't mean staying the same, but means being true to your values and growth?"

- **Historical Perspective**: "Think about ways you've already grown and changed. Are you less authentic now than you were in elementary school, or have you become more fully yourself?"

- **Multiple Authenticity**: "You're probably different with your friends than with your grandparents. Which version is the 'real' you? Maybe authenticity means having the flexibility to express different aspects of yourself appropriately."

The Social Identity Bridge

When peer relationships complicate change:

1. **Social Impact Assessment**: "How do you think your friends would react if you made these changes? What are your biggest concerns?"

2. **Relationship Evaluation**: "Which of your relationships support you growing and changing? Which ones seem to require you to stay exactly the same?"

3. **Authentic Relationship Building**: "What would it be like to have relationships where people appreciated you for growing and trying new things?"

4. **Gradual Introduction**: "How could you introduce small changes gradually so your friends get used to seeing different aspects of you?"

Case Study: Identity-Conscious Change in Action

Let's return to Alex, the class clown who wants to be taken more seriously:

Traditional Approach: "Alex, you need to stop joking around in class and start participating seriously. Your humor is preventing people from seeing your intelligence."

Identity-Conscious Approach:

Counselor: "Alex, I've noticed you have this amazing ability to help people feel comfortable and included through humor. That's actually a really valuable leadership quality. And you've also mentioned wanting people to recognize your intelligence. I'm wondering – is there a way to use both of those strengths?"

Alex: "What do you mean?"

Counselor: "Well, some of the most effective leaders and communicators use humor strategically – to make serious points more accessible, to help people relax enough to think clearly, to create connection before sharing important ideas. What would it look like if you experimented with using your humor as a bridge to sharing your thoughts on serious topics?"

Alex: "So like... still be funny, but also smart-funny?"

Counselor: "Exactly. You wouldn't be abandoning who you are – you'd be expanding it. What would smart-funny Alex look like in class?"

This approach honors Alex's core identity (humor as a social strength) while creating space for growth (intellectual contribution). He can experiment with change without feeling like he's betraying himself.

Developmental Timing and Identity Work

Identity development follows predictable patterns that affect change readiness:

Early Adolescence (11-14): Identity exploration is just beginning. Teens may resist changes that feel like they're locking them into permanent self-definitions. Emphasize experimentation and reversibility: "Let's try this and see how it fits."

Middle Adolescence (15-17): Peak identity exploration period. Teens are most open to change that feels connected to identity development but most resistant to change that threatens peer relationships. Focus on social integration strategies.

Late Adolescence (18-21): Identity consolidation begins. Teens become more open to changes that align with their emerging sense of direction and values. This is an optimal time for significant behavior changes that support long-term goals.

Identity and Cultural Context

Identity development doesn't happen in isolation – it's deeply influenced by cultural, family, and community contexts:

Cultural Identity Integration: For teens from minority or multicultural backgrounds, change processes may involve navigating multiple cultural identities. Changes that work in one cultural context might create conflicts in another.

Family Identity Roles: Many teens have established roles within their families (the responsible one, the athlete, the artist) that complicate change processes. Family system changes may be necessary to support individual teen changes.

Socioeconomic Identity Considerations: Teens from different socioeconomic backgrounds may face different identity-related barriers to change. Understanding these contextual factors is crucial for effective change support.

Gender and Sexual Identity Development: For teens exploring gender or sexual identity, other changes may feel secondary to or complicated by this primary identity development work.

Supporting Healthy Identity Development

Rather than seeing identity development as an obstacle to change, adults can support healthy identity formation in ways that enhance change capacity:

Identity Affirmation: Regularly acknowledge and appreciate positive aspects of teens' current identities. This creates security that enables growth.

Growth Mindset About Identity: Help teens understand that identity can be both stable and evolving. Strong identities aren't fixed – they're flexible and adaptive.

Value Clarification: Support teens in identifying their core values, which can serve as stable anchors during identity exploration and change processes.

Role Model Exposure: Introduce teens to diverse role models who demonstrate different ways of expressing similar core qualities or values.

Identity Narrative Work: Help teens develop coherent stories about their identity that include both stability and growth over time.

Understanding the relationship between identity development and change doesn't make change work easier – it makes it more realistic and ultimately more successful. When we honor teens' developmental need to construct a coherent sense of self while also supporting their growth, we create conditions where authentic, lasting change becomes possible.

This identity-conscious approach transforms how we understand teen "resistance." Instead of seeing obstinance or fear, we can recognize appropriate developmental caution about changes that might threaten their emerging sense of self. This understanding opens up new pathways for connection and growth.

The key insight: teens aren't just deciding whether to change their behavior – they're deciding whether to change their story about who they are. When we help them write new chapters that build on rather than replace previous chapters, change becomes not just possible but exciting.

Essential Takeaways

Working with identity-conscious change requires patience, creativity, and deep respect for the complexity of adolescent development. You're not just helping teens modify behaviors – you're supporting them through one of the most important psychological tasks of human development: figuring out who they are and who they want to become.

When change feels identity-consistent rather than identity-threatening, teens move from resistance to curiosity, from fear to excitement. That transformation creates the foundation for the practical work of change – which begins with shifting how parents and teens communicate about growth and possibility.

Part II: Parent Guide Section

Chapter 4: From Lectures to Conversations

Fifteen-year-old Jordan walks through the front door twenty minutes past curfew, and his father David is waiting in the living room. David has been rehearsing this conversation for the past hour, mentally organizing his points about responsibility, safety, and consequences. As Jordan tries to slip upstairs, David launches into what he considers a reasonable explanation of why curfews matter.

"Jordan, we need to talk. Do you understand how worried your mother and I get when you don't come home on time? We set these rules because we love you and want to keep you safe. When you break curfew, you're not just breaking a rule – you're showing disrespect for our family values. I was never allowed to come home late when I was your age, and it taught me responsibility. I need you to understand that actions have consequences, and if this continues..."

Three minutes into David's speech, Jordan's eyes have glazed over. He's nodding mechanically while mentally composing a text to his girlfriend about how his dad "doesn't get it." When David finishes and asks, "Do you understand?" Jordan mumbles "Yeah, sorry" and disappears to his room. David feels frustrated and unheard. Jordan feels lectured and misunderstood. Nothing has actually changed.

This scene plays out in homes across America every day. Well-meaning parents, armed with legitimate concerns and years of life experience, deliver carefully reasoned monologues to teenagers who respond with apparent compliance but internal resistance. The harder parents try to make their points, the more teens seem to shut down.

But what if the problem isn't teenage defiance or parental inadequacy? What if the issue is the fundamental structure of these interactions –

the assumption that change happens through information transfer rather than collaborative exploration?

The Lecture Trap

Parents naturally gravitate toward lecture-style communication because it feels logical and efficient. You have important information, your teenager needs to understand it, so you explain it clearly and thoroughly. This approach works well for teaching algebra or explaining how to change a tire. But when it comes to motivating behavioral change, lectures often backfire spectacularly.

Why Lectures Don't Work for Change:

Information Overload: The adolescent brain, already struggling to integrate emotional and rational information, becomes overwhelmed when presented with multiple complex points simultaneously. Instead of processing the content, teens' brains often shut down or switch to defensive mode.

Autonomy Threat: Lectures inherently position the parent as the expert and the teen as the student. For adolescents developmentally driven toward independence, this dynamic triggers automatic resistance regardless of the merit of the message.

Passive Reception: Lectures require teens to passively receive information rather than actively engage with it. Research in learning theory shows that passive information reception is the least effective way to promote understanding or behavior change (Deci & Ryan, 2000).

Emotional Disconnection: When parents focus on delivering content, they often miss the emotional undertones of the situation. Teens may comply with the surface message while the underlying emotional issues remain unaddressed.

Reactance Effect: Psychological reactance theory explains that when people feel their freedom is threatened, they automatically resist – even when the restricting message is reasonable (Brehm, 1966).

Lectures often trigger reactance because they implicitly communicate "you must think this way."

Understanding Parental Motivation to Lecture

Before exploring alternatives, it's important to understand why parents default to lecturing despite its ineffectiveness:

Anxiety Management: Lecturing helps parents feel like they're doing something productive about their concerns. When you're worried about your teenager's choices, delivering a comprehensive explanation feels like taking action.

Control Illusion: Lectures create an illusion of control. If parents can just find the right words, present information clearly enough, or make compelling enough arguments, surely their teens will see reason and change.

Parental Modeling: Many parents lecture because they were lectured to as children. Even if they didn't enjoy it, it feels like proper parenting because it's what they experienced.

Time Pressure: In busy family schedules, lectures feel efficient. Rather than engaging in lengthy back-and-forth conversations, parents try to convey important information quickly and comprehensively.

Fear-Driven Communication: When parents are scared about their teen's safety or future, they often communicate from anxiety rather than connection. Lectures feel like they address the urgency of parental concerns.

The Neurobiological Reality of Teen Information Processing

To understand why lectures fail with teenagers, we need to understand how their brains actually process information and make decisions:

Emotional Processing Priority: The adolescent limbic system processes emotional information before rational information reaches the prefrontal cortex. When teens feel lectured, their emotional brain interprets this as criticism or control before their rational brain can evaluate the content (Steinberg, 2013).

Social Context Sensitivity: Teen brains are hyperattuned to social dynamics and power relationships. Lectures automatically trigger social threat detection systems because they establish clear hierarchies that teens' brains interpret as challenges to their developing autonomy.

Narrative vs. Analytical Thinking: Adolescent brains often process information through narrative frameworks rather than analytical ones. They think in stories about identity, relationships, and social meaning rather than logical cause-and-effect chains.

Peer Reference Default: When receiving information from adults, teen brains automatically compare it to peer perspectives and social norms. If parental messages conflict with peer group values, teens' brains often default to protecting peer relationships.

Shifting from Information Delivery to Collaborative Exploration

The alternative to lecturing isn't permissiveness or avoidance – it's **collaborative conversation**. This approach treats teens as partners in problem-solving rather than recipients of wisdom.

Core Principles of Collaborative Conversation:

Curiosity Over Certainty: Instead of starting with conclusions, begin with genuine questions about your teen's perspective and experience.

Exploration Over Explanation: Rather than explaining what teens should think, explore what they do think and why.

Partnership Over Hierarchy: Position yourself as a consultant or collaborator rather than an authority figure delivering mandates.

Process Over Content: Focus on how you're communicating, not just what you're communicating.

Connection Over Correction: Prioritize maintaining relationship connection even when addressing concerning behaviors.

The LEARN Conversation Framework

Here's a practical structure for shifting from lectures to conversations:

L – Listen First: Begin every significant conversation by genuinely listening to your teen's perspective before sharing your own.

E – Explore Together: Ask questions that help both of you understand the situation more deeply.

A – Acknowledge Complexity: Recognize that most teen situations involve competing values, emotions, and pressures rather than simple right/wrong choices.

R – Reflect Understanding: Demonstrate that you've heard and understood your teen's point of view before introducing your own concerns.

N – Navigate Solutions: Work together to identify solutions that address both your concerns and your teen's needs.

Let's see how David's curfew conversation might look using this framework:

Traditional Lecture Approach: *David*: "Jordan, we need to talk about curfew. When you come home late, you're showing disrespect and making us worry. We have these rules for good reasons, and I need you to follow them. This can't happen again."

LEARN Conversation Approach:

Listen: *David*: "Hey Jordan, I noticed you came in a bit late tonight. What was going on?"

Jordan: "We just lost track of time. We were at Mike's and his mom made dinner and it would have been rude to leave."

Explore: *David*: "That sounds like you were in a tricky social situation. Tell me more about what happened."

Jordan: "Well, Mike's parents don't see him much because of their work schedules, so when his mom actually cooked dinner, she really wanted us all to stay and eat together. I knew I'd be late, but I didn't want to hurt her feelings."

Acknowledge: *David*: "Wow, that's actually a pretty complex situation. You were trying to balance being respectful to Mike's family with following our family rules."

Reflect: *David*: "So you weren't just hanging out ignoring curfew – you were trying to navigate competing social expectations. That makes sense why you felt stuck."

Navigate: *David*: "I appreciate that you were being thoughtful about Mike's family. And I also need you to understand that when you're late, Mom and I genuinely worry about your safety. How could we handle this kind of situation differently next time?"

Notice how this approach gathers information, acknowledges complexity, and invites collaboration rather than delivering conclusions.

Common Conversation Mistakes and How to Avoid Them

Mistake #1: Fake Questions That Are Really Statements

Wrong: "Don't you think it would be better if you studied before watching TV?" (This is a lecture disguised as a question)

Right: "I'm curious about your thoughts on when the best time to study might be."

Mistake #2: Immediate Problem-Solving

Wrong: Jumping straight to solutions without understanding the teen's perspective

Right: Spending significant time exploring the situation before moving toward solutions

Mistake #3: Invalidating Teen Logic

Wrong: "That doesn't make any sense" or "You're not thinking clearly"

Right: "Help me understand your thinking on this" or "I can see how you came to that conclusion"

Mistake #4: Bringing Up Past Mistakes

Wrong: "This is just like when you..." or "You always..."

Right: Focusing on the current situation and future solutions

Mistake #5: Emotional Flooding

Wrong: Sharing all your fears, frustrations, and concerns at once

Right: Sharing one primary concern and gauging your teen's capacity for the conversation

Practical Conversation Starters

Instead of launching into explanations, try these conversation openers:

For Academic Issues:

- "I'm noticing some changes in your grades. What's your experience been like in school lately?"

- "Help me understand what's working and what's challenging for you academically right now."

For Social Concerns:

- "I've been wondering how things are going with your friends. What's the social scene like for you these days?"

- "I'm curious about your perspective on the friend situation you mentioned."

For Rule-Breaking:

- "I want to understand what happened from your point of view."

- "Walk me through your thinking on this decision."

For Future Planning:

- "What are you thinking about for next year?"

- "How do you see this situation playing out?"

For Emotional Support:

- "You seem like you've got a lot on your mind lately. What's it like being you right now?"

- "I'm wondering how you're processing everything that's been happening."

Managing Your Own Emotional Reactions

The biggest obstacle to collaborative conversation is often parental anxiety, frustration, or fear. When you're worried about your teenager, it's natural to want to download all your concerns immediately. But managing your own emotional state is crucial for effective communication.

Before Important Conversations:

Check Your Emotional Temperature: Am I feeling calm and curious, or anxious and controlling? If you're emotionally flooded, wait until you can approach the conversation from a more centered place.

Clarify Your Goal: Am I trying to control my teen's thinking, or genuinely understand their perspective? Be honest about whether you want a conversation or just compliance.

Consider Timing: Is this the right time for both of you? Teens are often more receptive to serious conversations when they're not rushing to school or coming down from social stress.

Prepare for Surprises: Your teen's perspective might be completely different from what you expect. Can you stay curious even if their viewpoint challenges your assumptions?

When Conversations Get Difficult

Even with the best intentions, conversations with teenagers can become heated, emotional, or stuck. Here are strategies for navigating challenging moments:

If Your Teen Shuts Down:

- "I can see this conversation isn't working for you right now. What would help?"

- "It seems like I'm coming across in a way I don't intend. Can you help me understand what's happening for you?"

If You Start Lecturing:

- Stop mid-sentence and restart: "I'm realizing I'm doing all the talking. I really want to hear your thoughts on this."

- "I'm falling into lecture mode. Can we back up and start with your perspective?"

If Emotions Run High:

- "We're both getting pretty heated. Should we take a break and come back to this?"

- "I can see we both care a lot about this. Let's slow down and try to understand each other."

If Your Teen Says "I Don't Know":

- "That's totally fair. This is complicated. What part of it feels clearest to you right now?"

- "Sometimes 'I don't know' means 'I'm not ready to talk about this.' Is that what's happening, or is it genuinely confusing?"

Building Conversation Skills Over Time

Shifting from lectures to conversations is a skill that develops with practice. Don't expect perfect collaborative discussions immediately – both you and your teen are learning new ways to communicate.

Start Small: Practice collaborative conversation techniques with low-stakes topics before tackling major issues.

Model Curiosity: Show genuine interest in your teen's thoughts about movies, music, friends, or current events. This builds comfort with sharing perspectives.

Share Your Own Thinking Process: Occasionally share how you think through decisions or handle challenges. This models that adults don't have all the answers and continue learning.

Ask for Feedback: "How did that conversation feel for you?" or "What would help these discussions work better?"

Celebrate Good Conversations: Acknowledge when you and your teen have productive discussions. This reinforces the value of collaborative communication.

Case Study: Sarah and Her Screen Time Struggles

Seventeen-year-old Sarah has been staying up until 2 AM on her phone, then struggling to wake up for school. Her mother Lisa is frustrated and worried about Sarah's sleep, grades, and general wellbeing.

Traditional Lecture Approach: *Lisa*: "Sarah, this phone situation has gotten out of hand. You're staying up way too late, you can barely get up in the morning, and your grades are suffering. Screen time before bed is terrible for sleep, and you're developing really unhealthy habits. I think we need to establish some clear boundaries. No phones in bedrooms after 10 PM, and maybe we should look into some apps that limit your usage. This is affecting your health and your future."

Sarah: *Rolls eyes* "Mom, everyone has their phones at night. You don't understand what my life is like. I need to stay connected with my friends."

Lisa: "Your friends will survive if you don't text them all night. Sleep is more important than social media."

Sarah: *Shuts down* "Whatever. Can I go now?"

Collaborative Conversation Approach:

Lisa: "Sarah, I've noticed you've been pretty tired in the mornings lately, and I'm wondering what's going on."

Sarah: "I just have trouble falling asleep."

Lisa: "Tell me more about that. What's it like when you're trying to go to sleep?"

Sarah: "Well, I get in bed, but then I start thinking about everything – school stuff, friend drama, college applications. My brain won't shut off. So I go on my phone to distract myself."

Lisa: "That makes sense. It sounds like your mind is processing a lot at bedtime. What happens when you're on your phone?"

Sarah: "Usually I'm texting with Emma about whatever drama happened that day, or watching TikToks. It helps me stop thinking about stressful stuff."

Lisa: "So your phone is kind of serving as stress relief and connection with Emma. I can understand why that would be appealing when your brain is spinning with worries."

Sarah: "Exactly! It's not just mindless scrolling. I'm actually dealing with real stuff."

Lisa: "That makes a lot of sense. And I'm also noticing that you're pretty exhausted in the mornings, which seems like it's making your days harder. Have you noticed that connection?"

Sarah: "Yeah, I'm definitely tired. But I don't know how else to handle all the stress and stay connected with my friends."

Lisa: "So you're in a tough spot – you need ways to manage stress and maintain friendships, and you also need sleep to function well during the day. What ideas do you have for addressing both of those needs?"

This conversation opens up collaborative problem-solving rather than creating a power struggle. Sarah feels heard and understood, while Lisa's concerns about sleep are acknowledged without being dismissed.

The Long-Term Benefits of Conversational Communication

When parents consistently choose conversation over lecture, several important things happen:

Increased Teen Openness: Adolescents become more willing to share their real thoughts and experiences when they know they won't be met with immediate judgment or lengthy explanations.

Enhanced Problem-Solving Skills: Teens develop better critical thinking abilities when they're regularly asked to reflect on situations and generate solutions rather than being told what to do.

Stronger Parent-Teen Relationships: Collaborative communication builds mutual respect and trust, creating a foundation for continued connection as teens mature into adults.

More Effective Change: When teens participate in identifying problems and generating solutions, they're more invested in following through with changes.

Improved Family Communication: Other family members often adopt more collaborative communication patterns when parents model this approach consistently.

What This Means for Your Family

Making the shift from lectures to conversations requires patience with yourself and your teenager. You're changing communication patterns that may have been established for years, and that doesn't happen overnight.

Start by paying attention to when you feel the urge to lecture. Notice the emotions driving that urge – usually anxiety, frustration, or fear. Instead of immediately acting on those emotions, take a breath and ask yourself: "What do I really want to know about my teen's experience right now?"

Remember that your teenager is developing critical thinking skills, emotional regulation, and decision-making abilities. Collaborative conversations support that development, while lectures can inadvertently undermine it.

The goal isn't to eliminate all parental guidance or boundaries. It's to deliver that guidance in ways that respect your teen's developing autonomy while maintaining connection and influence.

Moving Forward

This foundational shift in communication style creates the groundwork for addressing specific challenges that families face with teenagers. When you've established a pattern of collaborative conversation, it becomes possible to tackle complex issues like balancing school, activities, and screen time without immediately triggering teen defensiveness or parent-teen power struggles.

The communication skills you're developing serve as the foundation for all other aspects of motivational work with teenagers – because real change happens through relationship and understanding, not through information transfer and compliance.

Chapter 5: The Schedule Struggle

Every Sunday night, the Martinez family sits down to review the upcoming week. Sixteen-year-old Sofia has AP Chemistry lab reports due Monday, a history presentation Wednesday, soccer practice Tuesday and Thursday, a game Saturday, plus her part-time job Friday evening. She also wants to maintain her social connections, get enough sleep, and somehow fit in college application work that's been looming over everything.

Her parents, Elena and Miguel, look at Sofia's packed schedule with a mixture of pride and concern. They want to support her academic success and extracurricular commitments, but they're watching their daughter become increasingly stressed, snappy, and exhausted. When they suggest she might need to drop an activity or reduce her work hours, Sofia becomes defensive: "Everyone else manages to do everything. I can't fall behind."

Meanwhile, Sofia's 14-year-old brother Carlos seems to live in a completely different universe. He'll spend three hours playing video games, then panic about homework at 10 PM. When his parents try to help him create a schedule, he agrees enthusiastically but never follows through. "I'll start being more organized tomorrow," he promises repeatedly, but tomorrow never comes.

Sound familiar? The schedule struggle is one of the most common sources of family tension during adolescence. Parents see teens either overcommitting to the point of burnout or undercommitting to the point of academic failure. Traditional approaches often backfire – rigid scheduling feels controlling to teens seeking autonomy, while complete freedom can lead to chaos and stress.

But what if the solution isn't about finding the perfect schedule? What if it's about helping teens develop **internal motivation** for balance and **personal systems** that align with their individual needs, learning styles, and values?

Understanding the Teenage Relationship with Time

Before jumping into scheduling solutions, it's crucial to understand how adolescent brains experience and process time differently than adult brains:

Present-Moment Bias: The developing prefrontal cortex struggles with future-oriented thinking and long-term planning. Teens genuinely experience difficulty connecting current actions with future consequences, making traditional time management approaches feel abstract and irrelevant (Steinberg, 2013).

Variable Energy Patterns: Adolescent circadian rhythms shift naturally toward later bedtimes and wake times. Most teens are biologically programmed to feel alert later in the evening and struggle with early morning cognitive demands (Carskadon et al., 2004). Fighting this biological reality often creates unnecessary scheduling conflicts.

Emotional Time Distortion: When teens are engaged in activities they enjoy or that feel socially important, their perception of time becomes distorted. Three hours gaming with friends might feel like 30 minutes, while 30 minutes of homework might feel like three hours.

Identity-Based Activity Prioritization: Teens don't just schedule activities – they schedule identity expressions. Soccer isn't just exercise; it might represent athletic identity, social belonging, and college planning simultaneously. Understanding this helps explain why teens resist dropping activities that adults see as "just" time commitments.

Social Schedule Synchronization: Teen scheduling isn't individual – it's deeply social. Their preferred timing for activities, homework, and social connection often revolves around peer availability rather than optimal personal productivity patterns.

The Mythology of Perfect Balance

Much of the scheduling advice targeted at teenagers assumes that perfect balance is both possible and desirable. This creates unrealistic expectations and unnecessary guilt for both teens and parents.

The All-Things-Equally Myth: The idea that teens should give equal attention to academics, extracurriculars, social life, family time, and self-care simultaneously sets everyone up for failure. Real life involves seasons of different focus and temporary imbalances.

The Productivity Optimization Myth: Adult productivity systems often emphasize maximum efficiency and output optimization. But teenagers are still developing executive function skills, emotional regulation, and identity clarity. Expecting adult-level productivity from developing brains is unrealistic and potentially harmful.

The External Schedule Imposition Myth: Many parents believe that if they can just create the right schedule for their teen, everything will fall into place. But externally imposed schedules often fail because they don't account for teen autonomy needs, individual learning patterns, or intrinsic motivation.

The Future-Self Motivation Myth: Traditional scheduling advice assumes teens will be motivated by long-term goals and future benefits. But adolescent brains are designed to prioritize immediate rewards and present-moment experiences.

A Different Approach: Values-Based Scheduling

Instead of starting with time management techniques, begin with helping teens identify what matters most to them and why. When scheduling decisions align with personal values, teens are more likely to sustain their commitments even when challenges arise.

The Values Exploration Process:

Step 1: Life Area Identification Help teens identify the major areas of their lives: academics, relationships, health, creativity, service, spirituality, future planning, etc. Don't impose categories – let them define what matters to them.

Step 2: Current vs. Desired Reality For each life area, explore two questions:

- "How much time and energy are you currently giving to this area?"

- "How much time and energy would you ideally like to give to this area?"

Step 3: Value Conflict Recognition Help teens recognize where their values create conflicts: "I value academic excellence AND social connection AND athletic achievement AND adequate sleep. When these compete for time, how do I decide?"

Step 4: Seasonal Prioritization Instead of trying to balance everything equally all the time, help teens think in seasons: "This semester, academics need to be my top priority because of AP exams. Next summer, I want to focus more on relationships and creativity."

Step 5: Implementation Alignment Once values and priorities are clear, scheduling becomes about alignment rather than obligation: "Given that academics are my priority this semester, what schedule would best support that value?"

Let's see how this might work with Sofia, our overcommitted student:

Traditional Approach: "Sofia, you're doing too much. You need to drop either soccer or your job so you can focus on school and get more sleep."

Values-Based Approach:

Parent: "Sofia, I can see you're juggling a lot right now. Help me understand what each of these activities means to you."

Sofia: "Well, soccer is huge for me. It's not just a sport – it's where my closest friends are, and I'm hoping for a college scholarship. My job isn't just about money; I'm saving for college, and I like feeling independent. And obviously school matters for college too."

Parent: "So soccer represents friendship, college opportunities, and athletic identity. Work represents independence and college preparation. School represents college preparation too. I can see why they're all important to you."

Sofia: "Exactly! That's why I can't just drop something."

Parent: "That makes sense. And I'm also noticing you seem really stressed and tired lately. What's your experience been with managing all of this?"

Sofia: "Honestly, it's really hard. I feel like I'm always behind on something. But I don't want to give anything up."

Parent: "What if we think about this differently? Instead of dropping activities, what if we looked at how to make your current commitments more sustainable? What would that look like?"

This approach honors Sofia's values while opening space for creative problem-solving rather than forcing elimination of meaningful activities.

Individual Differences in Schedule Management

Not all teenagers struggle with scheduling in the same ways. Understanding individual differences helps tailor approaches to each teen's specific needs:

The Overcommitter: Like Sofia, these teens take on too much because they see multiple activities as essential to their identity or future goals. They need help with prioritization and boundary-setting rather than motivation.

The Undercommitter: Like Carlos, these teens struggle with initiation and follow-through. They often have good intentions but lack systems for translating intentions into consistent action.

The Perfectionist Scheduler: These teens create elaborate planning systems but become paralyzed when reality doesn't match their perfect plans. They need help with flexibility and self-compassion.

The Chaos Embracer: These teens resist all scheduling attempts and seem to thrive on last-minute pressure. They need help finding structure that doesn't feel controlling.

The Social Scheduler: These teens organize their lives primarily around social connections and peer activities. They need help integrating other priorities without sacrificing relationships.

The Seasonal Motivator: These teens have periods of high engagement followed by periods of complete disengagement. They need help creating sustainable rhythms rather than constant high intensity.

Practical Scheduling Strategies for Different Types

For Overcommitters:

Priority Matrix Development: Help teens create a matrix of activities based on two criteria: personal importance and external requirement. This helps them see which activities are chosen versus imposed.

Energy Management Over Time Management: Focus on when they have the most energy for different types of activities rather than trying to fit everything into arbitrary time slots.

Strategic Saying No: Practice phrases and decision-making frameworks for evaluating new opportunities without automatic yes responses.

Stress Signal Recognition: Help teens identify early warning signs that they're overextended and create systems for scaling back before reaching burnout.

For Undercommitters:

Micro-Commitment Building: Start with very small, achievable commitments and gradually build capacity. Success breeds motivation more than motivation breeds success.

Environmental Design: Change physical and digital environments to make desired behaviors easier and undesired behaviors harder.

Social Accountability: Use peer connections and social commitments to create external structure that supports internal goals.

Interest-Based Entry Points: Connect required activities to teens' existing interests rather than treating them as separate obligations.

For Perfectionist Schedulers:

Good Enough Planning: Help teens create "good enough" plans that allow for flexibility and imperfection while still providing structure.

Buffer Time Integration: Build buffer time into schedules so that when things take longer than expected, the entire plan doesn't collapse.

Plan B Development: Create backup plans for when primary schedules don't work, reducing anxiety about schedule disruption.

Process Over Outcome Focus: Celebrate consistent effort and learning from schedule adjustments rather than perfect execution.

The Technology Integration Challenge

Modern teens must navigate scheduling in a digital world with constant connectivity, social media pressures, and device-based distractions. This requires different strategies than pre-digital approaches to time management:

Digital Distraction Management: Instead of eliminating technology, help teens create intentional relationships with their devices. This might include app usage awareness, notification management, and designated device-free times.

Social Media Reality Checks: Help teens recognize how social media creates unrealistic impressions of others' schedules and achievements. Everyone posts highlights, not the full reality of struggles and failures.

Online Learning Optimization: Many teens now balance in-person and online learning environments. This requires different focus strategies and schedule management approaches than traditional classroom-only education.

Virtual Social Connection: Teen social lives often happen across multiple digital platforms with different timing expectations. Help them think intentionally about which digital relationships deserve immediate responses and which can wait.

Family System Considerations

Teen scheduling doesn't happen in isolation – it affects and is affected by entire family systems:

Parental Modeling: Teens absorb parental attitudes toward time, balance, and priorities through observation more than instruction. Parents who constantly complain about being busy or who never model downtime send powerful messages about scheduling values.

Family Rhythm Integration: Individual teen schedules need to work within family rhythms and logistics. This requires negotiation and compromise rather than complete individual autonomy.

Sibling Comparisons: Different teens in the same family often have very different scheduling strengths and challenges. Avoid comparing siblings or applying the same systems to teens with different temperaments and needs.

Cultural and Economic Factors: Family scheduling is influenced by cultural values about achievement, independence, and family responsibility, as well as economic realities about work schedules, transportation, and activity costs.

Case Study: The Johnson Family's Screen Time Negotiation

The Johnson family is struggling with screen time management for their 15-year-old daughter Maya and 13-year-old son Tyler. Maya spends hours on social media but maintains good grades, while Tyler's gaming interferes with homework and sleep.

Traditional Approach: "We're implementing family screen time rules. No devices during homework time, no devices after 9 PM on school nights, and everyone gets two hours of recreational screen time per day."

Collaborative Approach:

Parent: "We've been having ongoing conflicts about screen time, and I don't think our current approach is working for anyone. I'd like to understand each of your perspectives and see if we can find something that works better."

Maya: "I don't think it's fair to have the same rules for Tyler and me. I keep up with my responsibilities, but he doesn't."

Tyler: "Gaming is how I connect with my friends! And I do get my homework done eventually."

Parent: "So Maya, you feel like you've demonstrated you can manage screen time responsibly, and Tyler, you feel like gaming is important for your friendships. Both of those make sense. And I'm concerned about homework getting done thoroughly and everyone getting enough sleep. What ideas do you have for addressing all of these concerns?"

Maya: "What if we each created our own screen time plan based on our individual situations, but we check in weekly to see how it's working?"

Tyler: "Could I have more gaming time on weekends if I finish homework earlier during the week?"

Parent: "Those are interesting ideas. Let's each think about what we need and what we're willing to try, and see if we can create individual agreements that work for our family."

This approach treats each teen as an individual while maintaining family values and parental boundaries.

Building Executive Function Skills

Rather than managing teens' schedules for them, the goal is helping them develop internal executive function skills that will serve them throughout life:

Planning Skills: Help teens break large projects into smaller steps, estimate time requirements realistically, and create backward planning from deadlines.

Initiation Skills: Support teens in developing personal systems for starting tasks they've been avoiding, including environmental cues, accountability partners, and motivation strategies.

Organization Skills: Work with teens to develop organization systems that match their thinking style and life patterns rather than imposing adult-preferred systems.

Time Awareness Skills: Help teens develop better awareness of how long activities actually take them versus how long they think activities will take.

Flexibility Skills: Support teens in developing resilience when schedules don't work as planned and skills for adjusting plans without abandoning goals entirely.

Self-Monitoring Skills: Teach teens to notice their own energy patterns, productivity cycles, and stress signals so they can make informed scheduling decisions.

When Professional Support is Needed

Sometimes scheduling struggles indicate underlying issues that require professional attention:

Learning Differences: Teens with ADHD, dyslexia, or other learning differences may need specialized strategies for time management and executive function.

Anxiety or Depression: Mental health challenges can significantly impact motivation, energy, and time perception. Professional support may be necessary before scheduling strategies can be effective.

Perfectionism: Severe perfectionism that interferes with completion of tasks or causes significant distress may require therapeutic intervention.

Family System Issues: When scheduling conflicts reflect deeper family communication or boundary issues, family therapy might be more helpful than individual scheduling strategies.

Creating Sustainable Family Rhythms

The most effective approach to teen scheduling often involves creating family rhythms that support individual needs while maintaining connection and shared values:

Weekly Family Check-ins: Regular conversations about upcoming schedules, potential conflicts, and support needs help prevent last-minute crises and create opportunities for collaborative problem-solving.

Flexible Routine Development: Establish family rhythms that provide structure without rigidity – like designated homework time that can shift based on daily needs, or weekly family meals that rotate timing based on everyone's schedules.

Individual and Family Goal Alignment: Help teens see how their individual scheduling decisions affect family functioning, and help families adjust expectations based on teens' developmental needs and individual differences.

Celebration of Balance: Notice and appreciate when family members make good scheduling decisions or support each other's time needs. This reinforces positive patterns without creating pressure for perfection.

The goal isn't perfect schedules or the elimination of all time-related stress. The goal is helping teens develop internal motivation for balance, personal systems that match their individual needs, and family communication patterns that support both autonomy and connection.

When parents approach scheduling as collaborative problem-solving rather than rule enforcement, teens develop better decision-making skills and feel more ownership over their choices. This foundation becomes crucial when addressing more complex challenges like risk behaviors, where the stakes are higher and the need for teen buy-in is essential.

What This Means for Your Family

Start by examining your own relationship with time and balance. Are you modeling the kind of schedule management you want your teen to develop? Are you creating family rhythms that support everyone's needs, or are you trying to force individual solutions onto family systems?

Remember that learning to manage competing priorities is a critical life skill that takes years to develop. Your teenager's scheduling struggles aren't signs of failure – they're normal parts of developing executive function, identity clarity, and personal values.

Chapter 6: Risk Behaviors

Seventeen-year-old Marcus comes home from a party with bloodshot eyes and the unmistakable smell of marijuana clinging to his clothes. His mother, Patricia, has been waiting up, her mind racing through worst-case scenarios she's read about in parenting articles. Her first instinct is to launch into a lecture about the dangers of drugs, the legal consequences, and how disappointed she is in his choices.

But Patricia pauses. She thinks about the conversations they've been having lately – the ones where she's been trying to listen more and lecture less. She takes a deep breath and says, "Hey Marcus, how was the party? You look pretty tired."

Marcus freezes, expecting the interrogation he's prepared for. When it doesn't come, he finds himself actually talking: "It was okay. Kind of weird, actually. Everyone was smoking, and I felt like I had to, but I didn't really like it. Made me feel paranoid and stupid."

This moment – this choice Patricia made to approach her son with curiosity rather than judgment – opens a door that lecturing would have slammed shut. It's the difference between pushing teens toward secrecy and creating space for honest conversation about the complex realities they face.

Risk behaviors during adolescence aren't anomalies or signs of moral failure. They're predictable aspects of brain development, identity exploration, and social navigation. The question isn't whether teens will encounter situations involving substances, relationships, and safety decisions – it's whether adults will respond in ways that support good decision-making or drive risky behavior underground.

Understanding the Teenage Risk Landscape

The adolescent brain is literally designed to seek novel experiences and push boundaries. This isn't a design flaw – it's an evolutionary feature that historically helped young people separate from their families, explore new territories, and develop the independence necessary for adult survival (Steinberg, 2013).

Neurobiological Risk Factors:

Reward System Hypersensitivity: During adolescence, dopamine receptors in the brain's reward system multiply rapidly, making teens more sensitive to potentially rewarding experiences than children or adults. This means the potential "high" from risky behaviors feels more compelling to teenage brains (Galván, 2010).

Social Brain Activation: Areas of the brain associated with social acceptance and peer evaluation are hyperactive during adolescence. The social reward of fitting in with peers can literally override rational decision-making systems, especially when peers are present or imagined (Chein et al., 2011).

Prefrontal Cortex Development: The brain's "CEO" – responsible for impulse control, consequence prediction, and rational decision-making – doesn't fully mature until the mid-twenties. Teens aren't just choosing to ignore consequences; their brains are genuinely less capable of integrating long-term thinking with immediate desires.

Emotional Regulation Challenges: The limbic system, which processes emotions and stress, develops faster than the prefrontal cortex that regulates it. This "maturational imbalance" means teens feel emotions more intensely while having fewer tools for managing those feelings appropriately.

These neurobiological realities don't excuse dangerous behavior, but they do explain why traditional scare tactics and rational arguments often fail with teenagers. When adults understand that teen brains are operating under different rules, they can adjust their approaches accordingly.

The Spectrum of Risk Behaviors

Risk behaviors exist on a spectrum from normal developmental exploration to genuinely dangerous activities. Understanding this spectrum helps adults respond proportionally rather than treating all risks equally:

Normative Risk-Taking: Trying new activities, pushing social boundaries, experimenting with identity, staying out late, minor rule-breaking. These behaviors serve important developmental functions and are engaged in by most adolescents.

Moderate Risk Behaviors: Occasional alcohol use, sexual experimentation, driving with friends, academic rule-bending, social media oversharing. These behaviors require attention and conversation but aren't necessarily signs of serious problems.

High-Risk Behaviors: Regular substance use, unprotected sex, reckless driving, self-harm, criminal activity, dangerous social media challenges. These behaviors pose genuine threats to safety and future opportunities and require immediate intervention.

Crisis-Level Behaviors: Suicidal ideation, severe substance abuse, dangerous eating behaviors, involvement with violence, sexual exploitation. These situations require professional intervention and safety planning.

The key insight: not all risky behaviors require the same response. A teen who tries alcohol at a party needs a different intervention than a teen who's drinking daily to cope with depression. Understanding these distinctions helps adults respond appropriately rather than either overreacting to normal exploration or underreacting to genuine dangers.

Approaching Sensitive Topics Without Judgment

The way adults initiate conversations about risk behaviors often determines whether teens will engage honestly or shut down completely. Judgmental approaches – even well-intentioned ones – typically backfire by triggering teen defensiveness and secrecy.

The Judgment Trap: When adults approach risk conversations with predetermined conclusions about what teens "should" think or do, teens immediately sense this and shift into defensive mode. They stop sharing real information and start managing impressions, which eliminates any chance of genuine influence.

Creating Judgment-Free Conversations:

Start with Curiosity: Begin with genuine questions about the teen's experience rather than statements about what they did wrong. "Help me understand what happened" works better than "I can't believe you did that."

Separate Behavior from Identity: Address specific actions without attacking the teen's character. "That was a risky choice" is different from "You're being irresponsible."

Acknowledge Complexity: Recognize that most risk situations involve competing pressures and values rather than simple right/wrong decisions. "That sounds like a complicated situation" validates the teen's experience.

Validate Underlying Needs: Identify and acknowledge the legitimate needs that risky behaviors might be attempting to meet. "It makes sense that you wanted to fit in with the group" doesn't excuse dangerous behavior but recognizes human motivation.

Express Care Without Condition: Make it clear that your concern comes from love and care for their wellbeing, not from judgment about their choices. "I'm worried because I care about you" is more effective than "I'm disappointed in you."

Let's see how this might work with a common scenario:

Judgmental Approach: "I found vaping supplies in your backpack. We've talked about this before. Vaping is dangerous, it's expensive, it's against school rules, and it's illegal at your age. You're grounded until you can prove you're making better decisions."

Curious Approach: "I found a vape in your backpack and I'm wondering what's going on. Can you help me understand your experience with this?"

The second approach is much more likely to lead to honest conversation about peer pressure, stress management, curiosity, or whatever factors are actually driving the behavior.

Harm Reduction vs. Abstinence Conversations

One of the most challenging aspects of discussing risk behaviors with teens involves balancing safety with realistic expectations. Abstinence-only approaches often fail because they don't acknowledge the complex realities teens actually face.

Understanding Harm Reduction: Harm reduction recognizes that some teens will engage in risky behaviors regardless of adult preferences. Instead of focusing exclusively on preventing the behavior, harm reduction aims to minimize the potential negative consequences.

This doesn't mean condoning dangerous activities or abandoning values. It means acknowledging reality and working to keep teens as safe as possible within that reality.

Abstinence-Focused Conversation Examples:

- "You should never drink alcohol until you're 21."
- "The only safe sex is no sex."
- "Just say no to drugs."
- "You shouldn't be at parties where there's drinking."

Harm Reduction-Informed Conversation Examples:

- "I hope you'll choose not to drink, and if you do find yourself in a situation with alcohol, here's how to stay safer..."

- "I'd prefer you wait to have sex, and if you do become sexually active, let's talk about protection and consent..."
- "I don't want you using drugs, and if you're ever in a situation where you feel pressured or unsafe, call me no matter what."
- "I'd rather you not go to parties with drinking, and if you do go, let's talk about how to handle difficult situations..."

When Harm Reduction Makes Sense:

High-Risk Teens: Teens who are already engaging in risky behaviors despite abstinence messages need harm reduction strategies to stay safer while hopefully working toward better choices.

Realistic Developmental Expectations: Some experimentation is developmentally normal. Harm reduction acknowledges this while minimizing dangers.

Trust Building: When teens know they can talk honestly about their experiences without automatic punishment, they're more likely to ask for help when they need it.

Crisis Situations: When teens are in immediate danger, harm reduction focuses on safety first and behavior change second.

When Abstinence Messages Are Important:

Clear Family Values: Parents have the right and responsibility to communicate their values clearly, even when using harm reduction approaches.

Legal and Safety Boundaries: Some behaviors (driving under the influence, illegal activities) require clear abstinence messages because the consequences are too severe for harm reduction approaches.

Young Adolescents: Younger teens may benefit more from clear abstinence messages, with harm reduction conversations becoming more relevant as they mature.

Individual Teen Factors: Some teens respond better to clear boundaries and expectations rather than nuanced harm reduction approaches.

Practical Strategies for Different Risk Behaviors

Substance Use Conversations:

Opening the Conversation: "I'm curious about your experiences with alcohol/marijuana/other substances. What have you observed at school or with friends?"

Exploring Motivations: "What do you think draws people to try substances? What have you heard from friends about their experiences?"

Discussing Risks Realistically: Share factual information about risks without exaggerating or using scare tactics. Teens often know when adults are being dishonest, which undermines credibility.

Harm Reduction Strategies: If a teen is already using substances, focus on reducing harm: avoiding driving, staying with trusted friends, knowing what they're consuming, recognizing signs of dangerous situations.

Family Values Integration: "Our family values health and making thoughtful decisions. How do those values apply to these situations?"

Relationship and Sexual Behavior Conversations:

Creating Safety for Discussion: "I want you to know that you can talk to me about relationships and sexuality. I might not always love what you tell me, but I'll always love you and want to help you stay safe."

Exploring Relationship Values: "What do you think makes a healthy relationship? What are your thoughts about respect, consent, and communication in relationships?"

Discussing Pressure and Decision-Making: "How do you handle situations where someone wants you to do something you're not sure about? What strategies work for you?"

Safety Planning: Whether teens are sexually active or not, they need information about consent, protection, and resources for getting help if needed.

Digital Safety and Social Media Risks:

Understanding Their Digital World: "Help me understand how you and your friends use social media. What are the positive aspects? What's challenging about it?"

Discussing Online Risks: Explore cyberbullying, sexting, privacy issues, and online predators in age-appropriate ways.

Digital Citizenship Values: "How do our family values about respect and kindness apply to online interactions?"

Creating Safety Plans: Establish agreements about sharing information, reporting concerning contacts, and managing social media conflicts.

Case Study: The Miller Family's Substance Use Conversation

Sixteen-year-old Emma Miller was caught drinking at a school dance. Her parents, Jennifer and Robert, need to address both the immediate situation and their ongoing concerns about Emma's choices.

Traditional Punitive Approach: "Emma, we're extremely disappointed. You broke school rules, you broke our trust, and you put yourself in danger. You're grounded for a month, and we're taking your phone. We've told you before that drinking is dangerous and illegal. This behavior has to stop immediately."

Collaborative Harm Reduction Approach:

Jennifer: "Emma, we know about what happened at the dance, and we'd like to understand the situation better. Can you walk us through what happened?"

Emma: "I didn't plan to drink. Sarah brought vodka and everyone was trying it, and I felt like I'd be weird if I didn't."

Robert: "So you felt social pressure to participate, even though it wasn't something you planned to do."

Emma: "Yeah, and honestly, I didn't like it. It tasted awful and made me feel sick."

Jennifer: "It sounds like you learned something about your own preferences from this experience. And we're concerned about the risks – both the immediate safety risks and the fact that you could have gotten in serious trouble with school."

Emma: "I know. I felt scared when they called everyone's parents."

Robert: "We need to talk about consequences because there were some serious rule violations here. And we also want to help you think about how to handle these situations differently in the future. What ideas do you have?"

Emma: "Maybe I could text you if I'm in a situation where I feel pressured? And I definitely don't want to feel that sick again."

Jennifer: "We appreciate that you're being honest with us about what happened. Let's talk about strategies for peer pressure situations, and let's also be clear about what the consequences will be for this incident."

This approach addresses the behavior while maintaining connection and creating opportunities for learning rather than just punishment.

Setting Boundaries: When and How

Even within collaborative, non-judgmental approaches, parents need to set and maintain appropriate boundaries around risk behaviors. The key is setting boundaries that are clear, enforceable, and connected to values rather than arbitrary power assertions.

Effective Boundary Setting Principles:

Values-Based Boundaries: Connect rules to family values and safety concerns rather than arbitrary authority. "We have a curfew because we value your safety and we worry when we don't know where you are" is more effective than "Because I said so."

Collaborative Development: When possible, involve teens in developing family rules and consequences. They're more likely to follow agreements they helped create.

Clear and Specific: Vague rules create confusion and conflict. "Be responsible" is less effective than specific agreements about communication, safety check-ins, and consequence frameworks.

Enforceable and Realistic: Don't make rules you can't or won't enforce. Empty threats undermine all future boundary-setting attempts.

Natural Consequences: When possible, let consequences flow naturally from choices rather than imposing arbitrary punishments. Loss of car privileges for drinking and driving makes sense; loss of social media for drinking doesn't.

Repair and Learning Focus: Consequences should emphasize learning and relationship repair rather than punishment for its own sake.

Boundary Setting Examples:

Substance Use Boundaries:

- "Our expectation is that you won't use alcohol or drugs. If you find yourself in a situation where you feel unsafe, call us and we'll come get you with no questions asked in that moment."

- "If we discover you've been using substances, we'll need to have a conversation about safety planning and there will be consequences related to activities where substance use might occur."

Relationship Boundaries:

- "We expect you to treat yourself and others with respect in relationships. We're here to support you and answer questions."

- "Physical intimacy is a big decision with real consequences. We want you to feel comfortable talking to us about these topics."

Safety Boundaries:

- "We need to know where you are and who you're with. This isn't about not trusting you – it's about being able to help you if something goes wrong."

- "Driving is a privilege that comes with serious responsibilities. Any unsafe driving choices will result in loss of driving privileges."

When Professional Help is Needed

Sometimes risk behaviors indicate underlying issues that require professional intervention. Parents need to recognize when family conversations and boundaries aren't sufficient.

Signs That Professional Help May Be Needed:

Escalating Risk Patterns: Risky behaviors that increase in frequency or severity despite family interventions.

Multiple Risk Behaviors: Teens engaging in several high-risk behaviors simultaneously often need professional assessment.

Underlying Mental Health Issues: Depression, anxiety, trauma, or other mental health concerns often drive risk behaviors.

Family System Issues: When family conflicts, communication patterns, or other systemic issues contribute to teen risk behaviors.

Legal Consequences: Involvement with law enforcement, school disciplinary actions, or other formal consequences may require professional support.

Impact on Functioning: When risk behaviors significantly interfere with school, relationships, or daily functioning.

Safety Concerns: Any behaviors that pose immediate threats to the teen's or others' safety require professional intervention.

Supporting Teens Through Risk Situations

When teens do encounter risk situations – whether by choice or circumstance – adult responses can either support better decision-making or drive teens toward more dangerous choices.

In-the-Moment Support:

Stay Calm: Your emotional reaction in crisis moments teaches teens whether they can come to you with problems or need to handle them alone.

Focus on Safety First: Address immediate safety concerns before discussing behavior choices or consequences.

Gather Information: Understand what happened before deciding how to respond.

Avoid Shame and Blame: Focus on problem-solving and learning rather than expressing disappointment or anger.

Follow Through Consistently: Once you've established how you'll handle these situations, follow through consistently so teens know what to expect.

Long-Term Support Strategies:

Regular Check-ins: Create ongoing opportunities for teens to discuss their experiences and concerns without waiting for crises.

Skill Development: Help teens develop decision-making, communication, and coping skills that reduce their likelihood of engaging in dangerous behaviors.

Social Support: Support teens in developing healthy peer relationships and activities that provide positive alternatives to risky behaviors.

Professional Resources: Connect teens with counselors, therapists, or other professionals when appropriate.

Family Relationship Investment: Strong family relationships are one of the best protective factors against risky behavior. Invest in your relationship with your teen consistently, not just during crisis moments.

Creating Family Safety Plans

Rather than waiting for risk situations to occur, proactive families create safety plans that establish how they'll handle challenging situations before they arise.

Family Safety Plan Components:

Communication Agreements: How will family members communicate about concerning situations? What are the expectations for check-ins, honesty, and information sharing?

Emergency Protocols: What should teens do if they find themselves in unsafe situations? Who should they call? How will parents respond?

Consequence Frameworks: What are the general principles that will guide consequences for risky behavior? How will consequences be determined?

Support Resources: What professional or community resources are available if needed? How will the family access these resources?

Values Clarification: What are the family's core values that guide decision-making about risk situations?

Regular Review: How often will the family review and update their safety plan as teens mature and circumstances change?

Moving Forward with Realistic Hope

Addressing teen risk behaviors requires balancing several competing needs: acknowledging developmental realities while maintaining safety expectations, building trust while setting boundaries, supporting autonomy while providing guidance.

The goal isn't to eliminate all risk from teenagers' lives – that's neither possible nor developmentally appropriate. The goal is to help teens develop internal motivation for safety, good judgment about risk assessment, and confidence that they can turn to trusted adults when they need support.

When families approach risk behaviors with curiosity rather than judgment, collaboration rather than control, and harm reduction alongside clear values, they create conditions where teens are more likely to make safer choices and more likely to seek help when they need it.

What This Approach Requires

This approach requires adults to manage their own anxiety about teen safety while staying connected and influential. It requires patience with the developmental process while maintaining appropriate expectations. Most importantly, it requires recognizing that the relationship you build with your teenager is the foundation for all other interventions.

The communication skills you develop for handling risk behaviors become essential when addressing mental health concerns – situations where the stakes may be even higher and the need for professional support more urgent.

Chapter 7: Mental Health Conversations

Fifteen-year-old Maya has always been an excellent student and involved daughter. But over the past few months, her parents, Priya and David, have noticed changes. Maya sleeps until noon on weekends, has stopped hanging out with friends, and her usually stellar grades are slipping. When they ask how she's doing, she says "fine" with increasing irritation.

Last week, Priya found Maya crying in her room. When asked what was wrong, Maya snapped, "Nothing! God, why does everyone keep asking me that?" Then she slammed her bedroom door. Priya stood outside, torn between respecting Maya's privacy and growing concern that something serious was happening.

David thinks Maya is just being a typical moody teenager and will outgrow whatever phase this is. Priya worries they're missing something important. Both parents struggle with questions that keep many families up at night: How do you tell the difference between normal adolescent struggles and genuine mental health concerns? When is professional help needed? And how do you bring up mental health without making things worse?

These aren't academic questions for today's families. **Adolescent mental health challenges have increased dramatically over the past decade**, with rates of depression and anxiety among teens rising significantly (Twenge et al., 2019). Yet many families still struggle to recognize mental health concerns, talk about them openly, or access appropriate support.

The good news? Early identification and intervention can make tremendous differences in teen mental health outcomes. Families don't need to become therapists, but they do need to become informed, supportive, and connected to professional resources when necessary.

Understanding Adolescent Mental Health

Mental health during adolescence operates differently than adult mental health. Teenage brains are still developing, identity formation is ongoing, and social pressures are intense. This creates unique vulnerabilities but also unique opportunities for positive intervention.

Developmental Mental Health Factors:

Neurobiological Vulnerability: The adolescent brain undergoes massive reorganization, particularly in areas responsible for emotion regulation and stress management. This neuroplasticity creates both vulnerability to mental health issues and opportunity for positive change (Casey et al., 2019).

Identity Formation Pressure: The core developmental task of adolescence – figuring out who you are – creates natural periods of confusion, anxiety, and mood fluctuation. Sometimes these normal identity struggles can trigger or mask more serious mental health concerns.

Social Brain Sensitivity: Teen brains are hyperreactive to social information, making peer relationships, social media interactions, and perceived social rejection particularly impactful on mental health (Blakemore, 2018).

Stress Response Changes: The adolescent stress response system is more reactive than adult systems, meaning teens often experience stress more intensely and recover more slowly from stressful events.

Hormonal Influences: Puberty brings dramatic hormonal changes that affect mood, sleep, appetite, and emotional regulation in ways that can mimic or contribute to mental health concerns.

Understanding these developmental factors helps families distinguish between normal adolescent challenges and concerning mental health symptoms. The key is recognizing patterns rather than isolated incidents, and intensity rather than simple presence of difficult emotions.

Recognizing When Teens Are Struggling

One of the biggest challenges parents face is distinguishing between typical teenage behavior and signs of mental health concerns. This difficulty is compounded by the fact that teens often mask their struggles or express them in ways adults don't immediately recognize.

Normal Adolescent Development vs. Mental Health Concerns:

Normal: Occasional moodiness, temporary friend conflicts, academic stress during challenging periods, sleep schedule changes, some risk-taking behavior, identity exploration.

Concerning: Persistent mood changes lasting weeks or months, social isolation from all friends and activities, dramatic academic decline, severe sleep disturbances, dangerous risk-taking, expressions of hopelessness or self-harm.

Red Flag Indicators That Warrant Professional Attention:

Mood and Emotional Changes: Persistent sadness, irritability, or mood swings that interfere with daily functioning. Expressions of hopelessness, worthlessness, or persistent guilt. Extreme mood changes that seem disconnected from circumstances.

Behavioral Changes: Significant changes in sleep patterns (sleeping much more or less than usual), appetite changes, loss of interest in previously enjoyed activities, social withdrawal from friends and family, decline in academic performance or attendance.

Physical Symptoms: Frequent headaches or stomachaches without medical cause, fatigue or loss of energy, frequent illness, significant weight changes.

Cognitive Symptoms: Difficulty concentrating or making decisions, memory problems, racing thoughts, persistent worry that interferes with functioning.

Social and Relationship Changes: Withdrawal from friends and family, conflict with previously close relationships, difficulty maintaining relationships, isolation from activities.

Risk Behaviors: Self-harm behaviors, substance use as coping mechanism, dangerous or impulsive behaviors, expressed thoughts of death or suicide.

The Importance of Pattern Recognition: Single incidents or brief periods of difficulty are usually not cause for alarm. Mental health concerns typically involve patterns of symptoms that persist over time and interfere with multiple areas of functioning.

Common Mental Health Challenges in Adolescence

Understanding specific mental health conditions helps families recognize symptoms and know when to seek professional help.

Depression in Adolescents:

Teen depression often looks different from adult depression. While adults might appear obviously sad or withdrawn, depressed teens might seem primarily irritable, angry, or unmotivated.

Common Signs: Persistent sad or empty mood, irritability or anger, loss of interest in activities, fatigue, sleep disturbances, appetite changes, difficulty concentrating, feelings of worthlessness or guilt, thoughts of death or suicide.

What Families Often Miss: Depression in teens can look like laziness, attitude problems, or normal teenage moodiness. The irritability and anger that often accompany teen depression can mask the underlying sadness.

Anxiety Disorders in Adolescents:

Anxiety is the most common mental health concern among teenagers, but it often goes unrecognized because it can present as perfectionism, social withdrawal, or physical complaints.

Common Signs: Excessive worry about multiple life areas, physical symptoms like headaches or stomachaches, avoidance of social situations or activities, perfectionism that interferes with functioning, panic attacks, sleep difficulties due to worry.

What Families Often Miss: High-achieving, well-behaved teens may have significant anxiety that's masked by their apparent success. Social withdrawal might be attributed to shyness rather than social anxiety.

Eating Disorders:

Eating disorders typically emerge during adolescence and can be life-threatening if not addressed early.

Common Signs: Significant weight changes, obsession with food, body image, or weight, avoiding eating in social situations, excessive exercise, mood changes related to eating or body image.

What Families Often Miss: Eating disorders aren't always about weight loss. They can involve binge eating, emotional eating, or exercise addiction. Athletes may be at particular risk.

Trauma and PTSD:

Teens may experience trauma from various sources: accidents, violence, abuse, witnessing traumatic events, or ongoing stressful situations like family conflict or community violence.

Common Signs: Re-experiencing traumatic events through nightmares or flashbacks, avoiding reminders of trauma, negative changes in thoughts and mood, changes in arousal and reactivity.

What Families Often Miss: Trauma responses can look like behavioral problems, academic difficulties, or social withdrawal rather than obvious trauma symptoms.

Opening Mental Health Conversations

Many families struggle with how to initiate conversations about mental health without making teens feel judged, pathologized, or more anxious.

Creating Safe Conversational Spaces:

Normalize Mental Health Discussions: Talk about mental health the same way you talk about physical health – as something everyone needs to pay attention to and take care of.

Use Observational Language: Start with what you've noticed rather than diagnoses or judgments. "I've noticed you seem pretty stressed lately" rather than "You're depressed."

Express Concern from Love: Make it clear that your concern comes from care, not criticism. "I'm bringing this up because I care about you and want to make sure you have support."

Ask Permission: "Would it be okay if we talked about how you've been feeling lately?" This gives teens some control over the conversation.

Avoid Minimizing: Don't try to fix problems immediately or suggest that teens should just think more positively. Listen and validate before problem-solving.

Conversation Starters for Different Situations:

General Check-ins: "How are you feeling about life in general these days?" or "What's been the most challenging part of your week?"

When You've Noticed Changes: "I've noticed you haven't been hanging out with friends as much lately. What's going on for you?"

When Teens Seem Overwhelmed: "You seem like you have a lot on your mind lately. Want to talk about what's going on?"

After Difficult Events: "That sounds like it was really hard. How are you processing what happened?"

When Physical Symptoms Appear: "You've had a lot of headaches lately. Sometimes stress can show up in our bodies. What do you think might be going on?"

Case Study: The Chen Family's Mental Health Journey

Sixteen-year-old Kevin Chen has always been a high achiever, but lately his parents have noticed concerning changes. He's staying up until 2 AM doing homework that used to take him half as long, he's stopped participating in family activities, and he had a panic attack during a recent math test.

Initial Conversation:

Mom: "Kevin, I've noticed you seem really stressed about school lately, and I'm wondering how you're feeling about everything."

Kevin: "I'm fine. Just busy with junior year stuff."

Dad: "The other day you mentioned feeling overwhelmed about the math test. Can you tell us more about what that was like?"

Kevin: "I don't know. I just... I couldn't breathe and my heart was racing. I felt like I was going to throw up or pass out. It was really scary."

Mom: "That sounds terrifying. Have you had experiences like that before?"

Kevin: "Kind of. Sometimes I wake up in the middle of the night feeling like that, thinking about all the stuff I have to do."

Dad: "It sounds like you're dealing with a lot of anxiety. That must be exhausting."

Kevin: "I guess. I thought I was just weak or something. Everyone else seems to handle this stuff fine."

Mom: "Anxiety is really common, especially with all the pressure you guys are under. It's not about being weak – it's about your brain and body responding to stress. Would you be open to talking to someone who specializes in helping people with anxiety?"

Kevin: "Like a therapist? I don't know... would that mean something's wrong with me?"

Dad: "Not at all. It would mean you're taking care of your mental health the same way you'd take care of a physical injury. We just want you to have support and tools to feel better."

This conversation normalizes Kevin's experience, validates his feelings, and introduces professional help as a normal, supportive resource rather than a last resort for serious problems.

Encouraging Professional Help Without Shame

One of the biggest barriers to teen mental health treatment is stigma – both societal stigma around mental health and family concerns about what seeking help means.

Reframing Mental Health Support:

Health Model vs. Pathology Model: Present therapy and mental health support as health maintenance rather than crisis intervention. "Just like we go to the doctor for physical check-ups, sometimes we need support for mental health."

Skill Development Focus: Frame therapy as learning skills and strategies rather than fixing problems. "A therapist can teach you tools for managing stress and anxiety."

Strength-Based Language: Emphasize that seeking help shows strength and self-awareness, not weakness. "It takes courage to ask for help when you need it."

Normalize Professional Support: Share examples of successful people who use therapy, mention that many people benefit from mental health support, and treat it as a normal part of healthcare.

Addressing Common Teen Concerns About Therapy:

"Nothing's wrong with me": "Therapy isn't just for when something's wrong. It's for when you want support, skills, or someone to talk to who isn't family."

"I don't want to talk to a stranger": "It can feel weird at first, but therapists are trained to help people feel comfortable, and you get to choose whether to continue after meeting them."

"My friends will think it's weird": "Actually, a lot of people your age go to therapy. You don't have to tell anyone if you don't want to, but you might be surprised how common it is."

"What if they tell my parents everything": Explain confidentiality rules and how therapists handle privacy with minors.

Practical Steps for Finding Mental Health Support:

Start with Your Pediatrician: Primary care doctors can provide initial mental health screening and referrals to specialists.

School Resources: Many schools have counselors or social workers who can provide support or referrals.

Insurance Provider Lists: Check with your insurance company for covered mental health providers.

Professional Referrals: Ask trusted healthcare providers, friends, or community members for recommendations.

Online Therapy Options: For some teens, online therapy feels more comfortable and accessible than in-person sessions.

Crisis Resources: Know how to access immediate help if needed – crisis hotlines, emergency rooms, or mobile crisis teams.

Supporting Treatment Engagement

Getting teens into therapy is often easier than keeping them engaged. Many adolescents attend reluctantly and may resist participating fully in treatment.

Strategies for Supporting Therapy Engagement:

Respect Teen Autonomy in Therapy: Allow teens to have private conversations with their therapists. Resist the urge to ask for detailed reports about sessions.

Focus on Outcomes, Not Process: Pay attention to whether therapy is helping your teen function better rather than trying to control what happens in sessions.

Address Practical Barriers: Make sure transportation, scheduling, and payment aren't barriers to consistent attendance.

Support Homework and Skills Practice: If therapists assign homework or skill practice, support these activities without taking over.

Be Patient with the Process: Mental health improvement often involves temporary setbacks and gradual progress rather than linear improvement.

Communication with Therapists: Maintain appropriate communication with your teen's therapist while respecting confidentiality boundaries.

When Therapy Isn't Working:

Give It Time: Most teens need several sessions to build rapport with therapists and start seeing benefits.

Address Specific Concerns: If your teen has specific complaints about therapy, help them communicate these to their therapist or consider whether a different therapist might be a better fit.

Consider Different Approaches: Some teens respond better to different therapeutic approaches – cognitive-behavioral therapy, family therapy, group therapy, or creative therapies.

Medication Considerations: For some mental health conditions, medication combined with therapy is more effective than therapy alone.

Family Support During Mental Health Treatment

While professional treatment is often necessary for teen mental health concerns, family support remains crucial for recovery and ongoing wellness.

Creating Supportive Home Environment:

Reduce Stress When Possible: Identify and minimize unnecessary stressors in your teen's environment while maintaining appropriate expectations.

Maintain Routines: Consistent daily routines support mental health recovery, but allow flexibility when teens are struggling.

Encourage Self-Care: Model and support healthy habits – regular sleep, physical activity, nutritious eating, and stress management.

Stay Connected: Continue investing in your relationship with your teen even when they're receiving professional help.

Avoid Over-Functioning: Don't take over responsibilities that your teen can handle independently, but provide support when needed.

Managing Family Stress: Teen mental health concerns affect entire families. Parents need support too – through their own therapy, support groups, or trusted friends and family members.

Sibling Considerations: Other children in the family may be affected by a sibling's mental health struggles. They need age-appropriate information, reassurance, and their own support.

Crisis Situations and Safety Planning

Sometimes teen mental health concerns escalate to crisis levels requiring immediate intervention. Families need to know how to recognize and respond to mental health emergencies.

Crisis Warning Signs:

Suicide Risk Factors: Direct statements about wanting to die, preoccupation with death, giving away possessions, sudden improvement in mood after a period of depression (which might indicate a decision to end life), increased risk-taking behavior.

Self-Harm Escalation: Increasing frequency or severity of self-harm behaviors, or self-harm behaviors that pose serious physical risk.

Psychotic Symptoms: Hearing voices, seeing things others don't see, paranoid thoughts, severe confusion or disorganization.

Severe Mood Episodes: Extreme depression that prevents basic functioning, manic episodes with dangerous behavior, or rapid cycling between extreme moods.

Crisis Response Steps:

Stay Calm: Your emotional state affects your teen's emotional state. Take care of your own anxiety so you can think clearly.

Ensure Immediate Safety: Remove means of self-harm if present, stay with your teen if they're at risk, call emergency services if there's immediate danger.

Use Crisis Resources: National Suicide Prevention Lifeline (988), crisis text lines, emergency rooms, or mobile crisis teams.

Follow Up Appropriately: Crisis intervention is just the first step. Follow up with appropriate professional care and safety planning.

Creating Family Safety Plans: Work with mental health professionals to create plans for managing future crisis situations, including warning signs, coping strategies, and emergency contacts.

Ongoing Mental Health Maintenance

Mental health isn't just about treating problems – it's about building ongoing wellness and resilience. Families can support teen mental health through everyday practices and attitudes.

Building Family Mental Health Practices:

Regular Check-ins: Create ongoing opportunities for family members to discuss how they're doing emotionally, not just practically.

Stress Management: Teach and model healthy stress management techniques – exercise, mindfulness, creative activities, social connection.

Emotional Literacy: Help teens develop vocabulary for emotions and practice identifying and expressing feelings appropriately.

Problem-Solving Skills: Support teens in developing skills for handling challenges independently while knowing when to ask for help.

Social Connection: Encourage healthy peer relationships and family connections that provide emotional support.

Meaning and Purpose: Help teens identify activities, relationships, and goals that provide meaning and motivation.

Physical Health Integration: Recognize connections between physical and mental health – sleep, nutrition, exercise, and medical care all affect mental wellness.

What This Means for Families

Mental health conversations with teenagers require the same principles that make other difficult conversations successful: curiosity over judgment, collaboration over control, and patience with the developmental process.

The goal isn't to become your teen's therapist or to solve all their problems. The goal is to create an environment where mental health is treated as a normal part of overall health, where teens feel comfortable seeking support when needed, and where families work together to promote wellness and resilience.

These conversations about mental health, like conversations about risk behaviors, require parents to manage their own anxiety while staying connected and supportive. The communication skills you've been developing – listening first, exploring together, acknowledging complexity – become essential when supporting teens through mental health challenges.

When families can talk openly about mental health, recognize concerning patterns, access professional support without shame, and maintain hope during difficult periods, they create conditions where teens can develop the emotional regulation skills, coping strategies, and support networks that serve them throughout life.

Section III: Professional Applications

Chapter 8: School-Based MI

Ms. Rodriguez stands outside her classroom door as students file in for third period American History. She notices Jamal dragging his feet, earbuds in, hood up despite the school's dress code. This is the fourth day this week he's arrived looking like he'd rather be anywhere else. His test grades have dropped from B's to D's over the past month, and yesterday he put his head down on his desk and didn't participate at all.

Ms. Rodriguez's first instinct is familiar to most educators: call Jamal out for the hood, remind him about classroom expectations, and maybe send him to the office if he doesn't comply. But she's been learning about different approaches to student engagement, and something tells her that traditional discipline isn't going to address what's really going on with Jamal.

After class, she approaches him differently: "Jamal, I've noticed you seem pretty disconnected from class lately. I'm wondering what's going on for you."

Jamal looks surprised by the genuine concern in her voice. Instead of the defensive response she expected, he says, "I don't know, Ms. R. This stuff just feels pointless. Like, when am I ever going to need to know about the Revolutionary War? I've got real problems to deal with."

This moment represents a choice point that every educator faces multiple times per day: respond with authority and curriculum requirements, or respond with curiosity about the student's experience. Ms. Rodriguez chooses curiosity, and that choice opens a door to understanding Jamal's perspective and finding ways to connect his "real problems" to his education.

School-based Motivational Interviewing isn't about lowering academic standards or eliminating structure. It's about recognizing that **student motivation is the foundation for all learning**, and that motivation comes from feeling heard, understood, and connected to something meaningful.

The School Environment Challenge

Implementing MI in schools requires adapting its principles to unique constraints and opportunities that don't exist in therapeutic or family settings:

Institutional Constraints: Schools operate within systems of standards, testing requirements, discipline policies, and time limitations that can feel incompatible with individualized, student-centered approaches.

Multiple Relationships: Educators work with 100+ students daily, making the deep, ongoing relationships that characterize traditional MI more challenging to develop.

Time Limitations: Class periods, administrative duties, and curriculum requirements leave limited time for extended MI conversations.

Authority Dynamics: Teachers inherently hold power over students through grading, discipline, and institutional authority, which can complicate the collaborative spirit of MI.

Group Settings: Most school interactions happen in group contexts where individual MI conversations are challenging.

Academic Focus: Schools primarily focus on cognitive learning, while MI addresses motivation and behavior change, requiring integration of both approaches.

But Schools Also Offer Unique Opportunities:

Daily Contact: Unlike therapists who see clients weekly, educators interact with students daily, providing multiple opportunities for brief MI interactions.

Natural Motivation Context: Academic challenges, peer relationships, and future planning are inherently motivational topics that students care about.

Developmental Relationships: Many students develop meaningful connections with educators that can serve as foundations for motivational work.

Real-World Application: School provides immediate opportunities for students to practice new behaviors and see results.

Adapting MI Principles for Educational Settings

Traditional MI was developed for clinical settings with individual clients. School-based MI adapts these principles for educational contexts:

From Individual to Brief Interactions: Instead of hour-long sessions, school-based MI happens in moments – a two-minute conversation after class, a brief check-in during passing periods, or a quick reflection during group work.

From Problem-Focused to Strength-Based: Rather than focusing primarily on problems students need to solve, school-based MI emphasizes student strengths, interests, and aspirations that can be connected to academic goals.

From Change Talk to Learning Talk: While clinical MI listens for "change talk" about problematic behaviors, school-based MI listens for "learning talk" – expressions of curiosity, interest, connection, and academic motivation.

From Resistance to Engagement: Instead of viewing student disengagement as resistance to overcome, school-based MI sees it as valuable information about mismatches between student needs and educational approaches.

From Individual Change to System Navigation: School-based MI helps students develop skills for navigating educational systems while also advocating for more responsive educational practices.

Academic Motivation and the Learning Brain

Understanding what motivates learning in adolescent brains helps educators apply MI principles more effectively:

Intrinsic vs. Extrinsic Motivation: Research consistently shows that intrinsic motivation (internal satisfaction, curiosity, mastery) leads to deeper learning than extrinsic motivation (grades, rewards, compliance). MI principles naturally support intrinsic motivation development (Deci & Ryan, 2000).

Autonomy and Academic Engagement: Students learn better when they feel some control over their learning process. This doesn't mean eliminating structure, but rather creating choices within structure and involving students in decision-making about their education.

Competence and Challenge: Students are motivated by tasks that are challenging but achievable. MI helps educators understand each student's current competence level and connect new learning to existing strengths.

Relatedness and Connection: Academic motivation increases when students feel connected to teachers, peers, and the material itself. MI's emphasis on relationship-building directly supports this need.

Purpose and Meaning: Adolescents are motivated by activities that feel meaningful and connected to their identity and future goals. MI helps students explore these connections explicitly.

Brief Interventions for Classroom Challenges

School-based MI happens primarily through brief interventions – short conversations that can shift student motivation and engagement:

The Two-Minute Check-In

Purpose: Build relationship and gather information about student experience

Process:

1. **Open with Curiosity**: "I noticed [specific observation]. What's your experience been like?"

2. **Listen for Understanding**: Focus on truly understanding the student's perspective rather than immediately problem-solving

3. **Reflect and Validate**: "It sounds like..." or "That makes sense because..."

4. **Identify Strengths**: "I can see that you..." (highlight something positive you've observed)

5. **Plant Seeds**: "I'm wondering if..." or "What would it look like if..." (introduce possibilities without pressure)

Example with Jamal: *Ms. Rodriguez*: "Jamal, I noticed you seem pretty disconnected from class lately. What's going on for you?"

Jamal: "I don't know. This stuff just feels pointless. When am I ever going to need to know about the Revolutionary War?"

Ms. Rodriguez: "So you're questioning the relevance of what we're studying to your actual life. That makes sense – you want your time to be spent on things that matter to you."

Jamal: "Exactly. I've got real problems to deal with."

Ms. Rodriguez: "I can see that you're someone who thinks seriously about what's important and what's worth your energy. That's actually a really valuable quality. I'm wondering if there might be connections between the stuff we're studying and the real problems you're thinking about that we haven't explored yet."

This brief interaction validates Jamal's perspective, identifies his strength (serious thinking about priorities), and opens possibilities without arguing or lecturing.

The Strength-Spotting Intervention

Purpose: Help students recognize their own capabilities and connect them to academic tasks

Process:

1. **Identify Specific Strengths**: Notice particular skills, efforts, or qualities students demonstrate

2. **Name Them Explicitly**: "I noticed that you..." (be specific about what you observed)

3. **Connect to Academic Goals**: "That skill could really help you with..."

4. **Invite Student Perspective**: "How do you see that strength showing up in other areas?"

Example: *Teacher*: "Marcus, I noticed that when we were discussing the debate about immigration policy, you were really good at seeing multiple perspectives. You didn't just argue for one side – you acknowledged the valid points that different people were making."

Marcus: "I guess. My family has different opinions about that stuff, so I hear all sides at home."

Teacher: "That's a really valuable skill – being able to understand different viewpoints even when you might not agree with them. That's exactly what good historians do, and it's what makes for strong writing too. I'm curious how you might use that skill in your research paper."

The Future-Focus Intervention

Purpose: Connect current academic tasks to student aspirations and goals

Process:

1. **Explore Student Goals**: "What are you hoping for after high school?" or "What kind of life do you want to build?"

2. **Listen for Values**: Pay attention to what matters to the student – independence, helping others, creativity, security, etc.

3. **Make Connections**: Help students see links between current academic work and their future goals

4. **Support Planning**: "What would help you move toward that goal?" or "What steps would make sense?"

Example: *Counselor*: "Destiny, I know you've been struggling with motivation in your math classes. Help me understand what you're hoping for after graduation."

Destiny: "I want to be a nurse. I want to help people and have a stable job that pays well."

Counselor: "Those are really meaningful goals – helping others and building financial security. What do you know about what it takes to become a nurse?"

Destiny: "I know you need to go to nursing school, and it's competitive to get in."

Counselor: "You're right – nursing programs are competitive, and they pay close attention to grades in science and math classes because nurses use that knowledge every day. They calculate medication dosages, monitor vital signs, understand how the body systems work. I'm wondering how your goal of helping people and building a stable career might connect to your math classes."

Engaging Reluctant Students

Every educator encounters students who seem disengaged, resistant, or unmotivated. Traditional approaches often focus on compliance and consequences, but MI offers alternative strategies:

Understanding Student Reluctance

Reluctance as Information: Instead of viewing student disengagement as a character flaw or discipline problem, MI treats it as valuable information about mismatches between student needs and current approaches.

Common Sources of Student Reluctance:

- **Academic Overwhelm**: Tasks feel too difficult or complex given current skill level

- **Relevance Questions**: Students can't see connections between academic work and their lives/goals

- **Relationship Issues**: Conflicts with teachers or peers affect engagement

- **External Stressors**: Problems at home, work, or in social relationships consume mental energy

- **Learning Differences**: Unidentified or unsupported learning challenges create frustration

- **Identity Conflicts**: Academic expectations conflict with peer group norms or family expectations

- **Previous Negative Experiences**: Past academic failures or trauma affect current willingness to engage

The OARS Approach in Schools

Open-Ended Questions:

- "What's your experience been like in this class?"

- "Help me understand what makes school feel worthwhile to you."

- "What would need to be different for you to feel more connected to this material?"

- "When do you find yourself most engaged in learning?"

Affirmations:

- "I can see that you care about doing things well."
- "You're asking really thoughtful questions about this topic."
- "It takes courage to admit when something is challenging."
- "I appreciate that you're being honest about your experience."

Reflections:

- "It sounds like you're feeling overwhelmed by all the requirements."
- "You're saying that this feels disconnected from your real life."
- "Part of you wants to succeed, and part of you feels like giving up."
- "You're wondering if the effort is worth it."

Summaries:

- "So on one hand, you want to do well because college matters to you. On the other hand, you're feeling frustrated because the work feels repetitive and you're not sure how it connects to your goals. You're trying to figure out how to stay motivated when things feel pointless."

Case Study: Engaging Marcus

Marcus is a junior who has stopped turning in assignments in his English class. His teacher, Mr. Peterson, uses MI principles to understand and address Marcus's disengagement.

Traditional Approach: "Marcus, you haven't turned in your last three assignments. This is affecting your grade and you're in danger of failing. You need to get caught up and start taking this class seriously."

MI Approach:

Mr. Peterson: "Marcus, I've noticed you haven't been turning in assignments lately, and I'm wondering what's going on for you."

Marcus: "I don't know. The essays feel stupid. Write five paragraphs about symbolism in a book that has nothing to do with my life."

Mr. Peterson: "So the assignments feel disconnected from your real experience and interests. That makes sense – you want your work to feel meaningful."

Marcus: "Yeah. Like, I get that reading is supposed to be important, but I don't see how writing about old books is going to help me with anything."

Mr. Peterson: "You're looking for connections between what we're doing in class and your actual goals. What are you hoping for after high school?"

Marcus: "I want to get into business. Maybe start my own company someday."

Mr. Peterson: "That's a great goal. Starting a business requires a lot of different skills. I'm curious – what do you think successful business owners need to be good at?"

Marcus: "Communication, I guess. Being able to convince people. Understanding what people want."

Mr. Peterson: "Those are exactly the skills we're working on in English class. Analyzing literature helps you understand human motivation – why people make the choices they do, what drives them, what they value. Writing helps you communicate your ideas clearly and persuasively. I'm wondering if there might be ways to connect your business interests to some of our assignments."

This conversation shifts Marcus from seeing English as irrelevant to seeing potential connections with his goals.

Working Within School System Constraints

One of the biggest challenges for educators interested in using MI is that schools often have systemic constraints that seem to conflict with MI principles:

Common System Constraints and MI Adaptations

Standardized Testing Pressure: *Constraint*: Pressure to raise test scores can lead to teaching-to-the-test approaches that feel disconnected from student interests.

MI Adaptation: Help students connect their personal goals to the skills measured by standardized tests. Use test preparation as an opportunity to develop general academic skills rather than just content knowledge.

Example: "I know the state test feels like a hoop to jump through. And the skills it measures – reading comprehension, analytical thinking, clear writing – those are actually skills you'll need for your goal of becoming a lawyer. Let's think about how preparing for this test can build skills you'll use throughout college and your career."

Rigid Curriculum Requirements: *Constraint*: Required curriculum content that may not align with student interests or seem relevant.

MI Adaptation: Find connections between required content and student interests, goals, or current events. Provide choices within requirements when possible.

Example: "I know we have to cover the Civil War for the state standards. I'm wondering what aspects of that time period connect to things you care about today – social justice, economic inequality, leadership during crisis, how ordinary people create change?"

Time Limitations: *Constraint*: Limited class time and multiple students make individual conversations challenging.

MI Adaptation: Use brief interventions, written reflections, and small group discussions to create opportunities for MI-style interactions.

Example: Use exit tickets with MI-style questions: "What was most meaningful about today's class for you?" or "How does today's topic connect to something you care about?"

Discipline Policies: *Constraint*: Zero-tolerance policies or rigid discipline systems that may not allow for MI approaches to behavior issues.

MI Adaptation: Use MI within existing systems when possible, and advocate for restorative approaches that align with MI principles.

Example: When required to issue consequences for behavior, combine them with MI conversations: "The policy requires this consequence, and I'm also wondering what was going on for you when this happened and how we can prevent similar situations in the future."

Building Administrative Support

Present Data: Share research on student engagement, intrinsic motivation, and academic outcomes associated with MI approaches.

Start Small: Begin with pilot programs, individual classroom implementations, or specific student populations before proposing school-wide changes.

Connect to School Goals: Frame MI approaches in terms of existing school priorities – improving test scores, reducing discipline referrals, increasing graduation rates.

Provide Professional Development: Offer training and support for staff interested in learning MI approaches.

Document Outcomes: Track changes in student engagement, behavior, and academic performance when using MI approaches.

Professional Development for Educators

Implementing school-based MI requires ongoing learning and practice for educators:

Core Competencies for School-Based MI

Relationship Building Skills:

- Creating psychological safety in classroom environments

- Demonstrating genuine curiosity about student experiences

- Building trust across cultural and generational differences

- Managing power dynamics inherent in teacher-student relationships

Communication Skills:

- Active listening techniques adapted for brief interactions

- Reflective responses that demonstrate understanding

- Open-ended questioning that promotes student self-reflection

- Summarizing skills that help students organize their thinking

Motivational Assessment Skills:

- Recognizing signs of intrinsic vs. extrinsic motivation

- Identifying student strengths and connecting them to academic tasks

- Understanding individual student goals and values

- Assessing readiness for different types of academic challenges

Intervention Skills:

- Adapting MI techniques for group settings

- Using brief interventions effectively within time constraints

- Integrating motivational work with academic instruction

- Knowing when to refer students for additional support

Training and Implementation Strategies

Gradual Implementation: Start by using MI principles with a small number of students or in specific situations before expanding to broader implementation.

Peer Learning: Create opportunities for educators to observe each other using MI techniques and provide mutual feedback and support.

Student Feedback: Regularly ask students about their experiences with different teaching and motivational approaches.

Reflective Practice: Use journals, peer discussions, or supervision to reflect on successes and challenges in implementing MI.

Ongoing Education: Participate in workshops, conferences, or coursework focused on motivational interviewing and student engagement.

School-Based MI

The goal of school-based MI isn't to transform schools into therapy centers or to eliminate academic rigor. The goal is to recognize that **motivation is the foundation for all learning** and to use evidence-based approaches to support student motivation alongside academic instruction.

When educators approach student disengagement with curiosity rather than frustration, when they connect academic work to student goals and values, and when they use their daily interactions to build motivation rather than just convey information, they create conditions where learning becomes more meaningful and effective for everyone involved.

School-based MI requires patience, practice, and systems thinking. Individual educators can begin implementing these approaches immediately in their own classrooms, but the greatest impact comes when entire schools create cultures that prioritize student motivation and engagement.

What This Means for Education

The communication skills and motivational approaches that work with individual students become even more powerful when applied to group settings. Understanding how to facilitate MI-informed group discussions, manage group dynamics, and harness peer influence for positive change extends the reach of these approaches beyond individual student relationships.

The foundation you're building through school-based MI – treating students as partners in their education, connecting learning to personal meaning, and using relationship as the vehicle for motivation – prepares you to work with groups of students who can support and motivate each other toward positive changes.

Chapter 9: Group MI

The after-school peer support group at Roosevelt High meets every Tuesday in Ms. Chen's classroom. Today, six students sit in a circle, ostensibly there to discuss stress management and academic success. But the energy in the room feels flat. Two students are on their phones, one is doing homework for another class, and the others look like they'd rather be anywhere else.

Traditional group facilitation might start with rules about phone use, followed by a structured discussion about predetermined topics. But Ms. Chen has been learning about group motivational interviewing, and she decides to try a different approach.

"Before we jump into anything formal," she says, "I'm curious what it's like for everyone to be here today. What brought you to group, and what are you hoping to get out of our time together?"

The question hangs in the air for a moment. Then Sophia, usually one of the quieter members, speaks up: "Honestly? I'm here because my mom thinks I need help with anxiety, but I'm not sure this is going to do anything."

Instead of defending the group or redirecting to the planned curriculum, Ms. Chen reflects: "So part of you is here because it matters to your mom, and part of you is skeptical about whether group discussions can actually help with anxiety. That makes sense – you want to spend your time on things that will actually make a difference."

Something shifts in the room. The phones disappear. Students start making eye contact. And suddenly, they're having a real conversation about what they actually want from this experience.

This moment illustrates the power of **Group MI** – adapting motivational interviewing principles to help groups of teenagers explore their own motivations, support each other's growth, and create collective energy for positive change.

The Unique Dynamics of Teen Groups

Group work with adolescents presents both tremendous opportunities and complex challenges that don't exist in individual MI conversations:

Peer Influence Amplification: During adolescence, peer relationships become primary sources of identity, belonging, and motivation. Groups can harness this natural peer influence for positive change, but they can also amplify resistance if not facilitated skillfully.

Social Brain Activation: Teen brains are hyperresponsive to social evaluation and peer acceptance. Group settings activate these systems intensely, creating both motivation for positive impression management and anxiety about judgment.

Identity Performance: Adolescents often perform different versions of themselves in different social contexts. Groups provide opportunities for teens to try on new identities with peer witness and support.

Collective Resistance: Groups can develop shared resistance to adult authority or change efforts. This collective resistance can be more powerful than individual resistance but also more amenable to peer influence interventions.

Modeling and Social Learning: Teens learn powerfully from observing peer behavior and decision-making processes. Groups provide natural opportunities for social learning and skill development.

Accountability and Support: Peer relationships can provide both motivation for change and ongoing support for sustaining new behaviors.

Adapting MI Principles for Group Settings

Traditional MI was developed for individual relationships, but its core principles can be adapted effectively for group work:

From Individual Change Talk to Collective Motivation

Individual MI listens for change talk from clients about their personal behavior changes. **Group MI** listens for expressions of collective values, shared goals, and group commitment to supporting each other's growth.

Example: *Individual Change Talk*: "I really want to improve my grades this semester." *Group Motivation Talk*: "We all seem to struggle with procrastination, and we could probably help each other figure out better strategies."

From Therapist Reflections to Peer Reflections

In individual MI, the practitioner provides reflections that demonstrate understanding. In group MI, facilitators teach group members to reflect each other's experiences, creating peer-to-peer understanding and validation.

Traditional Approach: *Facilitator*: "It sounds like you're feeling overwhelmed by college pressure."

Group MI Approach: *Facilitator*: "I heard Jamal sharing about feeling overwhelmed by college pressure. What did others hear, and how do you connect with that experience?"

From Individual Ambivalence to Group Exploration

Individual MI explores personal ambivalence about change. Group MI explores shared dilemmas and helps groups work through collective ambivalence about goals, norms, and behaviors.

Example: *Facilitator*: "I'm hearing that as a group, part of you wants to support each other in making healthier choices, and part of you worries about being judgmental or losing friendships if you speak up when someone's struggling. How do we navigate that tension together?"

From Practitioner Expertise to Collective Wisdom

Individual MI positions the client as the expert on their own experience. Group MI recognizes that groups collectively hold wisdom and solutions that no individual member (including the facilitator) possesses alone.

Traditional Approach: Facilitator provides information and solutions to group problems.

Group MI Approach: Facilitator helps the group access their collective knowledge and problem-solving capacity.

Facilitating Teen Groups Using MI Principles

Creating Psychological Safety

Before any meaningful group work can happen, members need to feel safe to share honestly without judgment or social risk:

Collaborative Ground Rules: Instead of imposing rules, engage the group in creating agreements about how they want to treat each other.

Facilitator: "What would need to be true in this group for you to feel comfortable sharing things that matter to you?"

Possible Responses: Confidentiality, no judgment, everyone gets to participate, no fixing or advice-giving unless requested, respectful disagreement is okay.

Address Power Dynamics: Acknowledge the facilitator's adult authority while minimizing hierarchical dynamics when possible.

Example: "I'm the adult in the room, which means I have certain responsibilities for safety and school policies. And I also want this to be a space where you have real influence over what we do and how we do it."

Normalize Differences: Create explicit permission for group members to have different perspectives, goals, and comfort levels.

Example: "Some of you might be here because you chose to be, others because someone suggested it, others because you're required to be here. All of those reasons are valid starting points."

The Group MI Opening Process

Individual Check-ins: Begin with brief individual sharing that helps group members connect with their own experiences and motivations.

Prompt: "Take a minute to think about what's going on in your life right now and what you're hoping for from our time together today. Who wants to start?"

Listen for Themes: As members share, listen for common experiences, shared values, or collective concerns that can become focus areas for the group.

Facilitator: "I'm hearing several people mention feeling stressed about college decisions, and also hearing that you care about supporting your friends. Those seem like areas where we might have good conversations as a group."

Explore Group Goals: Help the group identify what they want to accomplish together rather than imposing predetermined objectives.

Question: "Based on what people are sharing, what would make our time together feel worthwhile? What would you want to be different as a result of these conversations?"

Group Reflection Techniques

Popcorn Reflections: After someone shares, ask the group: "What did you hear?" Allow multiple brief reflections from different group members.

Feeling Checks: "How are people feeling about what Marcus just shared?" This helps process emotional content and builds empathy.

Value Identification: "What values do you hear behind what Destiny is saying?" This helps groups connect with shared values even when situations differ.

Strength Spotting: "What strengths did you notice in how Alex handled that situation?" Teaches group members to identify and affirm each other's capabilities.

Managing Group Dynamics and Resistance

Every teen group includes a range of personalities, motivations, and comfort levels. Skillful group MI helps manage these dynamics constructively:

Common Group Dynamics and MI Responses

The Dominator - Member who takes up excessive airtime or tries to control group discussions:

Traditional Response: Set limits or redirect privately.

Group MI Response: Reflect the person's engagement while creating space for others: "I can see this topic really matters to you, Marcus. I'm wondering what others are thinking about what you've shared."

The Silent Member - Person who participates minimally or seems disengaged:

Traditional Response: Call on them directly or encourage participation.

Group MI Response: Normalize different participation styles and offer low-pressure opportunities: "Some people process by talking, others by listening. Both are valuable. Quiet members, if something resonates with you, feel free to share, but no pressure."

The Skeptic - Member who questions the value of the group or challenges the process:

Traditional Response: Defend the group or minimize their concerns.

Group MI Response: Welcome skepticism as valuable information: "I appreciate your honesty about questioning whether this is helpful. Skepticism often means you care about not wasting time on things that don't work. What would need to happen for this to feel worthwhile to you?"

The Rescuer - Member who tries to fix everyone else's problems:

Traditional Response: Redirect to sharing their own experiences.

Group MI Response: Reflect the caring while protecting the group process: "I can see how much you care about helping others. That's a real strength. I'm also wondering what your own experience has been with the situation we're discussing."

Working with Collective Resistance

Sometimes entire groups develop resistance to the process, adult authority, or change efforts. Group MI approaches collective resistance as information about group needs:

Explore the Resistance: "I'm sensing some reluctance from the group today. Help me understand what's going on."

Validate Group Wisdom: "Groups often know when something isn't working for them. What would need to be different for this to feel more useful?"

Address Power Dynamics: "Sometimes groups feel like adults are trying to impose things on them. How are you experiencing our time together?"

Renegotiate the Process: "Based on what you're sharing, it sounds like we might need to adjust our approach. What ideas do you have?"

Case Study: The Academic Success Group

A group of eight juniors meets weekly to discuss academic motivation and college preparation. After three sessions, the energy is low and attendance is dropping. The facilitator, Mr. Davis, uses Group MI to address the resistance:

Traditional Approach: "I've noticed people seem disengaged and attendance is dropping. We need to recommit to the group process and focus on the important work of preparing for college."

Group MI Approach:

Mr. Davis: "I want to check in with everyone about how the group is feeling so far. I'm getting a sense that something isn't quite working, and I value your feedback about what you're experiencing."

Aisha: "No offense, but this feels like another class where adults tell us what we should want."

Carlos: "Yeah, and we all have different ideas about college anyway. Some of us aren't even sure we want to go."

Mr. Davis: "So you're experiencing this as adults imposing goals on you, and you're saying that group members actually have different perspectives about college and what you want for your futures. That's really valuable feedback."

Jessica: "I mean, I do want help with college stuff, but not like, generic advice. My situation is complicated."

Mr. Davis: "It sounds like you want support that's actually relevant to your individual situations rather than one-size-fits-all approaches. And Aisha and Carlos, you're pointing out that even the goal of college prep might not fit everyone in the group. What would need to be different for this group to feel genuinely helpful to each of you?"

Kevin: "What if we could talk about our actual situations instead of hypothetical college planning stuff?"

Aisha: "And what if people who aren't sure about college don't have to pretend they are?"

Mr. Davis: "Those sound like great suggestions. What I'm hearing is that you want this to be a space where you can explore your real questions about the future – whether that includes college or not – and where you can get support that's actually relevant to your individual situations. How would that work?"

This conversation transforms a failing group into one where members feel heard and are invested in creating something that meets their actual needs.

Peer Support and Accountability

One of the most powerful aspects of Group MI is how it harnesses natural peer influence for positive change:

Building Peer Support Systems

Teach Supportive Responses: Help group members learn to respond to each other in ways that build motivation rather than create defensiveness.

Less Supportive: "You just need to try harder in math." *More Supportive*: "It sounds like math is really frustrating right now. What's been most challenging about it?"

Create Accountability Partners: Help group members form supportive relationships that extend beyond group time.

Process: "Based on what people have shared today, who might be good accountability partners for each other? What kind of support would be most helpful?"

Normalize Setbacks: Help groups understand that change involves setbacks and that peer support includes helping each other navigate difficulties.

Example: "Everyone has weeks when their goals don't go as planned. How can we support each other during those times without being judgmental?"

Peer Accountability Without Judgment

Focus on Values, Not Behaviors: Help group members hold each other accountable to their stated values and goals rather than to specific behaviors.

Question: "You mentioned that independence is really important to you. How do you see your current choices supporting that value?"

Use Questions, Not Statements: Teach group members to use curious questions rather than judgmental statements when offering accountability.

Less Effective: "You're not following through on your goals." *More Effective*: "How are you feeling about your progress toward the goals you set?"

Celebrate Effort, Not Just Outcomes: Help groups recognize and affirm each other's efforts and learning, not just successful outcomes.

Example: "Even though the presentation didn't go how you planned, I noticed you prepared really thoroughly and you tried something that was scary for you."

Practical Group MI Techniques

The Values Exploration Circle

Purpose: Help group members identify and share their core values as foundation for motivation and decision-making.

Process:

1. **Individual Reflection**: Members spend 5 minutes writing about what matters most to them in life

2. **Pair Sharing**: Members share with partners and listen for values underlying their goals

3. **Group Sharing**: Pairs share one value they heard from their partner and why it seemed important

4. **Group Discussion**: "What do you notice about our collective values? Where do we have common ground?"

The Ambivalence Exploration

Purpose: Help groups work through collective ambivalence about goals or changes.

Process:

1. **Name the Ambivalence**: "It seems like as a group, part of you wants X and part of you wants Y."

2. **Separate Sides**: Have group members physically move to different sides of the room based on which side of the ambivalence they relate to most

3. **Explore Each Side**: Each side shares their perspective while the other side listens without responding

4. **Find Integration**: "How might we honor both sides of this dilemma?" or "What would a solution look like that addresses both concerns?"

The Collective Wisdom Process

Purpose: Access the group's combined knowledge and experience to address individual member challenges.

Process:

1. **Member Presents Challenge**: One group member shares a specific situation they're struggling with

2. **Group Listens**: Other members listen without immediately offering advice

3. **Reflective Questions**: Group members ask curious questions to understand the situation better

4. **Share Similar Experiences**: Members share their own experiences with similar challenges (not advice)

5. **Collective Brainstorming**: Group generates ideas together, with the presenting member deciding what feels most helpful

The Progress Celebration Circle

Purpose: Help group members recognize growth and maintain motivation for continued change.

Process:

1. **Individual Preparation**: Members think about one area where they've grown or changed since joining the group

2. **Sharing**: Each member shares their growth area without minimizing or qualifying their progress

3. **Peer Recognition**: Other group members reflect what they've observed about that person's growth

4. **Strength Identification**: Group helps each member identify personal strengths that contributed to their growth

5. **Forward Focus**: "What do you want to keep building on based on this progress?"

Special Considerations for Teen Groups

Developmental Appropriateness

Identity Exploration Support: Recognize that teen groups are spaces for identity development and experimentation. Create permission for members to try on different aspects of themselves.

Social Learning Emphasis: Take advantage of teens' natural tendency to learn from peer observation and modeling.

Future-Focus Integration: Help groups connect current experiences to future goals and aspirations without imposing adult timelines or expectations.

Autonomy Respect: Balance structure with choice, and adult guidance with teen self-determination.

Cultural Responsiveness

Multiple Perspectives: Actively welcome and explore different cultural perspectives within the group rather than assuming shared experiences.

Communication Style Awareness: Recognize that different cultures have different norms about self-disclosure, emotional expression, and group participation.

Family System Acknowledgment: Understand that teens' group participation may be influenced by family expectations, values, or constraints.

Intersectional Identity Recognition: Help groups address how multiple aspects of identity (race, gender, sexuality, class, religion) affect members' experiences and perspectives.

Crisis Management in Groups

Individual Crisis Support: Know how to provide individual support while maintaining group safety and process.

Group Trauma Response: Understand how traumatic events affecting one group member impact the entire group and how to facilitate group support.

Professional Boundaries: Maintain clarity about when group facilitation needs to include professional counseling or referral resources.

Safety Planning: Create clear protocols for handling disclosures of abuse, self-harm, or other safety concerns within group settings.

Building Sustainable Group Programs

Program Design Considerations

Flexible Duration: Consider both time-limited groups (8-12 sessions) and ongoing groups based on member needs and institutional constraints.

Mixed Motivation Accommodation: Design groups that can serve both voluntary participants and those attending due to external requirements.

Skill Building Integration: Combine MI principles with concrete skill development relevant to group goals.

Outcome Measurement: Track both individual member progress and group development indicators.

Facilitator Development

MI Training: Ensure facilitators have solid grounding in individual MI principles before adapting to group settings.

Group Dynamics Knowledge: Provide training in adolescent group development, stage models, and common group challenges.

Cultural Competence: Support facilitators in developing skills for working with diverse teen populations.

Self-Care Emphasis: Address the unique stresses of group facilitation and provide ongoing support for facilitators.

What This Builds Toward

Group MI with teenagers creates powerful opportunities for peer learning, mutual support, and collective motivation for positive change. When teens experience being truly heard by peers, when they practice supportive communication skills, and when they participate in groups that honor their autonomy while providing structure, they develop capacities that serve them throughout life.

The skills you develop in group settings – managing complex dynamics, facilitating difficult conversations, and supporting collective decision-making – become essential when working with teens in crisis situations where emotions run high and safety concerns require immediate attention.

Chapter 10: Crisis Moments

The text message arrives at 11:47 PM: "Ms. Johnson, I can't do this anymore. Everything is falling apart and I don't see the point."

Sarah Johnson, a high school counselor, stares at her phone. The message is from Tyler, a 16-year-old she's been working with who's been struggling with depression and academic pressure. Her mind races through protocols, risk assessments, and emergency procedures. But underneath the professional training, she feels the weight of this moment – a teenager reaching out in his darkest hour, and her response could make the difference between connection and crisis escalation.

In crisis moments, everything changes. The luxury of long-term relationship building disappears. The option for gradual exploration of ambivalence evaporates. Suddenly, you're dealing with acute emotional dysregulation, immediate safety concerns, and the need to make quick decisions while maintaining the human connection that makes healing possible.

This is where Motivational Interviewing is both most challenging and most crucial. Traditional crisis intervention often focuses on immediate safety and symptom management – essential functions that sometimes override relationship concerns. But MI principles offer something additional: ways to maintain human connection and support autonomy even during crisis moments.

Crisis MI isn't about replacing safety protocols or minimizing serious risks. It's about using MI principles to enhance crisis response – creating more effective de-escalation, better engagement with overwhelmed teens, and stronger foundations for ongoing support after the immediate crisis passes.

Understanding Teen Crisis States

Crisis moments in adolescence have unique characteristics that differ from both childhood and adult crises:

Neurobiological Intensity: The adolescent brain's maturational imbalance means that teens experience emotional crises more intensely than adults. Their limbic systems are highly reactive while their prefrontal cortex regulation systems are still developing (Casey et al., 2019).

Identity Threat Sensitivity: Because identity formation is the central developmental task of adolescence, situations that threaten teens' sense of self can trigger crisis responses disproportionate to the objective circumstances.

Social Context Amplification: Teen crises often involve peer relationships, social status, or perceived social rejection. The adolescent brain's sensitivity to social evaluation can turn interpersonal conflicts into existential crises.

Future Catastrophizing: Teens' developing capacity for abstract thinking can lead to catastrophic predictions about the future based on current difficulties. A failed relationship or academic setback can feel like evidence that their entire future is doomed.

Limited Coping Repertoire: Unlike adults who have decades of experience managing difficult emotions and situations, teens often have limited tools for handling intense stress, leading to feeling overwhelmed more quickly.

Authority Resistance During Distress: The developmental drive toward autonomy can make teens resistant to adult help even when they desperately need it, complicating crisis intervention efforts.

Understanding these developmental realities helps adults approach teen crises with appropriate expectations and strategies.

The Neuroscience of Crisis and Connection

When teenagers are in crisis, their brains shift into survival mode, affecting how they process information and respond to interventions:

Amygdala Hijack: During intense emotional states, the amygdala (threat detection center) can overwhelm the prefrontal cortex (rational thinking center), making logical reasoning difficult or impossible (LeDoux, 2015).

Cortisol Impact: Stress hormones released during crisis states impair memory formation, decision-making, and emotional regulation. This means teens in crisis may not remember conversations clearly or be able to think through solutions normally.

Social Connection as Regulation: The teen brain is particularly responsive to social connection as a form of emotional regulation. Feeling understood and supported can literally calm the nervous system and restore prefrontal cortex functioning.

Autonomy Threat Response: When teens perceive that adults are trying to control them during crisis moments, it can trigger additional stress responses that escalate rather than de-escalate the situation.

Safety Through Relationship: Research shows that perceived relational safety can be more calming to distressed teens than environmental safety measures, making the quality of adult response crucial.

These neurobiological realities suggest that crisis intervention approaches focusing solely on safety and symptom control may miss opportunities to activate the brain's natural recovery systems through connection and autonomy support.

De-escalation Through MI

Traditional de-escalation techniques focus on reducing emotional intensity and behavioral agitation. MI de-escalation adds relationship-based elements that can be more effective with adolescents:

The CALM Approach to Crisis MI

C - Connect Before Content Before addressing the crisis situation or offering solutions, establish genuine human connection through presence and understanding.

Traditional Approach: "Let's talk about what happened and figure out how to solve this problem."

MI Approach: "I can see you're really struggling right now. I'm here with you."

A - Acknowledge Without Minimizing Recognize the teen's emotional experience as valid without dismissing their pain or rushing to reassurance.

Avoid: "It's not as bad as you think" or "This will pass"

Instead: "This feels overwhelming right now" or "You're in a lot of pain"

L - Listen for Understanding Focus on truly understanding the teen's perspective and experience rather than immediately assessing risk or planning interventions.

Question: "Help me understand what this feels like for you right now."

Reflection: "It sounds like everything feels impossible and you don't see any way forward."

M - Maintain Hope and Agency Support the teen's sense of agency and possibility without minimizing the current crisis.

Statement: "Right now feels unbearable, and you have strength and resources that can help you get through this."

Crisis MI Conversation Example

Tyler's Crisis Text Response:

Ms. Johnson (calls Tyler): "Tyler, I got your text and I'm really glad you reached out. That took courage. Can you talk right now?"

Tyler: "I guess. I don't know what the point is though."

Ms. Johnson: "It sounds like you're feeling hopeless right now, like nothing you do makes a difference."

Tyler: "Exactly. I failed my chemistry test, my girlfriend broke up with me, and my parents are freaking out about college applications. I can't handle all of this."

Ms. Johnson: "So you're dealing with academic stress, relationship loss, and family pressure all at once. That's a lot for anyone to handle. No wonder you feel overwhelmed."

Tyler: "Everyone keeps telling me I need to try harder or think positive, but I'm already trying as hard as I can. It's not working."

Ms. Johnson: "You're already putting in maximum effort and still struggling, and then people suggest you should just try harder. That must feel incredibly frustrating and discouraging."

Tyler: "Yeah. Like, what's the point of trying if it doesn't matter?"

Ms. Johnson: "When you're already giving everything you have and it doesn't feel like enough, it makes sense that you'd question whether effort is worth it. That's a normal response to feeling overwhelmed."

Tyler: "I just don't know what to do anymore."

Ms. Johnson: "Right now, everything feels impossible and you can't see clear next steps. That's actually normal when someone is dealing with as much as you are. Your brain is overwhelmed, not broken."

Notice how Ms. Johnson validates Tyler's experience without minimizing his pain, reflects his feelings accurately, and normalizes his responses while maintaining implicit hope that the situation can change.

Using MI During High-Emotion Situations

High-emotion moments require adapted MI techniques that account for the teen's compromised cognitive capacity:

Simplify Communication

Short Sentences: Use brief, clear statements rather than complex explanations. *Example*: "You're in pain" instead of "I can see that you're experiencing significant emotional distress because of multiple stressors."

Immediate Present Focus: Stay focused on the present moment rather than exploring past causes or future implications. *Example*: "What do you need right now?" rather than "Let's think about how this pattern developed."

Concrete vs. Abstract: Use concrete language rather than abstract concepts. *Example*: "Your body feels tense and your thoughts are racing" rather than "You're experiencing anxiety."

Emotional Validation Techniques

Name the Emotion: Help teens identify and name their emotional experience. *Example*: "It sounds like you're feeling scared and angry and sad all at once."

Normalize Intensity: Acknowledge that intense emotions are normal responses to difficult situations. *Example*: "Most people would feel overwhelmed in your situation."

Separate Emotions from Actions: Help teens understand that feeling intense emotions doesn't mean they have to act on them. *Example*: "Feeling like you want to give up makes sense. Feeling that way doesn't mean you have to act on it right now."

Building Immediate Safety Through Connection

Physical Presence: When possible, offer physical presence or ask about who could be with the teen. *Question*: "Is there someone who could come be with you right now?"

Immediate Environment: Help teens identify what would make their immediate environment feel safer. *Question*: "What would help you feel a little safer right where you are?"

Breathing and Grounding: Use simple grounding techniques that involve the teen's choice and control. *Example*: "Would it help to take some slow breaths together, or would you prefer to do something else to help your body calm down?"

Safety Planning and Risk Assessment

Crisis MI must integrate safety planning and risk assessment while maintaining MI principles:

Collaborative Safety Assessment

Rather than doing risk assessment "to" teenagers, involve them in the assessment process:

Open Questions About Safety:

- "Help me understand how safe you're feeling right now."

- "What thoughts are going through your mind about hurting yourself?"

- "When you think about getting through tonight, what feels most challenging?"

Scaling Questions:

- "On a scale where 10 means you're definitely safe and 1 means you're in immediate danger, where are you right now?"

- "What would need to happen for that number to go up even one point?"

Resource Assessment:

- "Who in your life helps you feel safer when you're struggling?"

- "What has helped you get through really hard times before?"

- "What reasons do you have for staying safe right now?"

Collaborative Safety Planning

Traditional safety planning often involves adults creating plans for teenagers. MI safety planning involves teens in creating their own safety strategies:

Identifying Personal Warning Signs: *Question*: "What signs let you know when you're starting to feel this way?" *Follow-up*: "What would your friends or family notice about you when you're getting to this point?"

Developing Coping Strategies: *Question*: "What helps you feel even a little bit better when you're struggling?" *Follow-up*: "What could you do instead of hurting yourself when these feelings get intense?"

Building Support Networks: *Question*: "Who could you reach out to when you're feeling this way?" *Follow-up*: "What would make it easier for you to actually contact them?"

Professional Support Integration: *Question*: "What would need to be true about professional help for it to feel useful rather than just another burden?"

Case Study: Collaborative Crisis Planning

Maria's Self-Harm Crisis:

Maria, a 15-year-old, has been cutting herself and tells her school counselor that the urges are getting stronger and more frequent.

Traditional Safety Planning: *Counselor*: "We need to create a safety plan. When you feel like cutting, you should call the crisis hotline, remove sharp objects from your environment, and talk to your parents or me."

Collaborative MI Safety Planning:

Counselor: "I'm concerned about your safety, and I also want to create a plan that actually works for you. Help me understand what happens right before you cut yourself."

Maria: "Usually I'm feeling overwhelmed and angry, and cutting is the only thing that helps me feel better."

Counselor: "So cutting serves a real purpose for you – it provides relief when you're overwhelmed. That makes sense. I'm wondering what else might give you that sense of relief without hurting your body."

Maria: "I don't know. Nothing else works as well."

Counselor: "Cutting works really effectively for you right now. And I'm also wondering about your long-term goals for how you want to handle intense emotions. What would you want to be different about how you cope with overwhelming feelings?"

Maria: "I'd want to not need to hurt myself to feel better. But I don't know how to get there."

Counselor: "That's a meaningful goal – finding other ways to get relief when you're overwhelmed. What ideas do you have about small steps toward that?"

Maria: "Maybe I could try other things first before cutting? Like, give myself permission to cut, but try something else for like ten minutes first?"

Counselor: "That's a really thoughtful approach – not trying to eliminate cutting immediately, but creating space to try other strategies. What would you want to try during those ten minutes?"

This approach honors Maria's current coping strategy while supporting her autonomy in developing alternatives, making the safety plan more likely to be followed.

When MI Isn't Enough - Knowing Limits

MI principles enhance crisis intervention, but they don't replace professional judgment about when more directive interventions are necessary:

Clear Indications for Directive Intervention

Imminent Safety Threats: When teens are in immediate physical danger to themselves or others, safety takes precedence over collaboration.

Psychotic Episodes: When teens are experiencing breaks from reality, they may not be capable of collaborative decision-making and need immediate professional intervention.

Severe Intoxication: When substance use has impaired judgment to dangerous levels, immediate safety measures take priority.

Legal Requirements: When situations involve mandatory reporting requirements or legal interventions, these must be addressed regardless of MI principles.

Integrating Directive Care with MI Principles

Even when directive interventions are necessary, MI principles can enhance the process:

Explain Your Reasoning: Help teens understand why directive actions are necessary. *Example*: "I need to call your parents because you're talking about specific plans to hurt yourself. I know this isn't what you want, and I'm more concerned about your safety than about your preferences right now."

Maintain Respect: Continue to treat teens with dignity even when overriding their preferences. *Example*: "I'm making this decision for you right now, and it doesn't mean I don't respect your feelings or opinions about it."

Plan for Autonomy Return: Communicate that directive interventions are temporary and that collaborative approaches will resume as soon as safely possible. *Example*: "Right now I need to make decisions about your safety. As soon as you're safer, we'll go back to making decisions together."

Professional Support Integration

Crisis MI practitioners need clear protocols for when to involve additional professional support:

Mental Health Professionals: When teens need assessment for psychiatric conditions, medication evaluation, or ongoing therapy.

Medical Professionals: When physical health concerns accompany emotional crises.

Child Protective Services: When abuse or neglect concerns arise during crisis intervention.

Law Enforcement: When situations involve immediate threats to safety that require legal intervention.

Family Support Services: When family system issues contribute to or complicate teen crises.

Building Crisis Response Systems

Effective crisis MI requires systemic support rather than just individual practitioner skills:

Organizational Preparation

Training and Protocols: Ensure staff understand both MI principles and crisis intervention requirements.

Resource Networks: Develop relationships with mental health professionals, medical services, and family support resources.

Follow-up Systems: Create procedures for ongoing support after immediate crises are resolved.

Self-Care Support: Provide support for practitioners who regularly engage in crisis intervention work.

Community Integration

School-Community Partnerships: Build relationships between schools and community mental health resources.

Family Education: Help families understand crisis signs and response strategies.

Peer Support Programs: Train teens to recognize crisis signs in friends and know how to get help.

Prevention Focus: Use crisis experiences to identify and address underlying systemic issues that contribute to teen crises.

After the Crisis - Maintaining Connection

Crisis intervention doesn't end when immediate safety is secured. The relationships built during crisis moments can provide foundations for ongoing support:

Processing Crisis Experiences

Normalize Crisis Recovery: Help teens understand that recovering from crisis takes time and that setbacks are normal parts of the process.

Identify Learning: Explore what teens learned about themselves, their coping capacity, or their support systems during the crisis.

Celebrate Strength: Acknowledge the courage it took to reach out for help and the strength demonstrated by surviving the crisis.

Plan for Future Challenges: Use the crisis experience to develop better strategies for handling future difficulties.

Strengthening Support Systems

Relationship Repair: Help teens reconnect with family or friends who may have been affected by the crisis.

Professional Connections: Support transitions to ongoing mental health care or other professional support.

Skill Development: Connect teens with resources for developing better coping strategies and emotional regulation skills.

Meaning Making: Help teens integrate crisis experiences into their overall life narrative in ways that support growth rather than shame.

What Crisis Work Teaches

Crisis intervention with teenagers using MI principles reveals fundamental truths about adolescent development and human resilience. Teens in crisis haven't lost their capacity for wisdom, growth, or decision-making – they're temporarily overwhelmed by circumstances that exceed their current coping resources.

When adults can maintain faith in teens' fundamental competence even during crisis moments, when they can provide safety without eliminating autonomy, and when they can offer support without taking over, they create conditions where crisis becomes an opportunity for growth rather than just survival.

Chapter 11: Transition Planning

Eighteen-year-old Jasmine sits across from her guidance counselor, Mr. Martinez, surrounded by college brochures, scholarship applications, and career assessment results. It's February of her senior year, and everyone seems to have opinions about her future. Her parents want her to pursue pre-med because "doctors have job security." Her favorite teacher thinks she should study creative writing because "she has real talent." Her best friend is pressuring her to attend the same college so they can room together.

But when Mr. Martinez asks Jasmine what she wants, she stares at the ceiling and says, "I honestly have no idea. Everyone acts like this decision will determine my entire life, and I don't even know what I want to do next year, let alone forever. What if I choose wrong? What if I disappoint everyone? What if I disappoint myself?"

Jasmine's struggle represents one of the most challenging applications of MI principles: supporting teenagers through major life transitions without imposing adult timelines, expectations, or definitions of success. Transition planning conversations require helping teens explore their authentic interests and values while navigating family expectations, societal pressures, and their own developmental uncertainties.

Traditional transition planning often focuses on matching students to predetermined pathways – college, career, or trade school – based on academic performance and general interest assessments. But MI-informed transition planning recognizes that **the process of thoughtful decision-making is more important than any specific decision outcome**. The goal isn't to get teens to make perfect choices, but to help them develop skills for making authentic choices that align with their values and aspirations.

The Developmental Reality of Teen Transition Planning

Adolescent brain development creates unique challenges for transition planning that adults often underestimate:

Abstract Thinking Development: While teens can engage in some future-oriented thinking, their capacity to imagine detailed future scenarios and predict long-term consequences is still developing. Asking a 17-year-old to choose a career path assumes cognitive capabilities that may not be fully mature (Steinberg, 2013).

Identity Formation Timing: The primary developmental task of adolescence is identity exploration, not identity commitment. Pressuring teens to make premature commitments can actually interfere with healthy identity development (Marcia, 1980).

Experience Limitations: Most teens have limited real-world exposure to different career paths, college experiences, or life options. They're making major decisions based on theoretical knowledge rather than experiential understanding.

Peer Influence Integration: Teen decision-making is naturally influenced by peer relationships and social considerations. This isn't immaturity – it's developmentally appropriate social cognition that needs to be integrated into transition planning.

Family System Pressures: Adolescents are simultaneously individuating from their families while still being dependent on them. This creates complex dynamics around transition decisions that involve both autonomy development and family loyalty.

Understanding these developmental realities helps adults approach transition planning with appropriate expectations and support teens through decision-making processes that honor their developmental stage.

College and Career Conversations

Traditional college and career counseling often focuses on external criteria – grades, test scores, job market projections, and family resources. MI-informed approaches start with the student's internal experience and work outward to practical considerations:

Starting with Values and Interests

Values Exploration Questions:

- "When you imagine yourself as an adult, what kind of life do you want to be living?"

- "What matters most to you in how you spend your time?"

- "What kinds of problems do you care about solving?"

- "What environments help you feel energized and engaged?"

Interest Discovery Process: Rather than relying solely on interest inventories, help teens explore their authentic curiosity and engagement patterns:

- "Tell me about times when you've lost track of time because you were so engaged in something."

- "What topics do you find yourself reading about or watching videos about in your free time?"

- "When you help other people, what kinds of help do you most enjoy providing?"

- "What would you want to learn more about even if it wasn't required?"

Moving from Interests to Possibilities

Once teens have explored their values and interests, help them connect these internal experiences to external opportunities:

Possibility Generation: *Question*: "Based on what you've shared about valuing creativity and wanting to help people, what kinds of college programs or career paths might align with those values?"

Follow-up: "What other possibilities come to mind, even ones that might seem unrealistic right now?"

Information Gathering Support: *Traditional Approach*: Provide information about different options and let teens choose.

MI Approach: Support teens in actively seeking information that addresses their specific questions and concerns.

Question: "What would you most want to know about [specific option] to help you evaluate whether it might be a good fit?"

Follow-up: "How could you find out more about that? Who could you talk to or what could you experience that would give you better information?"

Case Study: Supporting Authentic Career Exploration

David's Engineering Pressure:

David is a high school senior with strong math and science grades. His father, an engineer, assumes David will pursue engineering. David has always been good at math, but he's not sure it's his passion.

Traditional Approach: *Counselor*: "Your grades in math and science are excellent, and engineering is a stable career field with good earning potential. Have you looked into different engineering programs?"

MI-Informed Approach:

Counselor: "David, you've got strong skills in math and science, and I'm wondering what your own experience has been with those subjects. What draws you to them, and what's your experience like when you're working on math or science problems?"

David: "I'm good at them, and they come easily to me. But honestly, I don't know if I enjoy them that much. I do well, but I don't get excited about them like some of my friends do."

Counselor: "So there's a difference between being good at something and being passionate about it. What do you get excited about? When do you feel most engaged and energized?"

David: "I really like working with people. I tutor younger kids in math, and I love seeing them understand concepts for the first time. And I've been volunteering at a community center, helping with after-school programs."

Counselor: "It sounds like you're drawn to helping others learn and grow. You value using your skills to support other people's development. How do you think about balancing those interests with your academic strengths?"

David: "I never thought about it that way. I guess I assumed I had to choose either math/science or working with people, not both."

Counselor: "What if you didn't have to choose? What possibilities come to mind when you think about combining your academic strengths with your interest in helping people learn and grow?"

David: "Maybe teaching? Or educational psychology? Or even engineering programs that focus on community development?"

Counselor: "Those all sound like possibilities worth exploring. What would help you learn more about whether any of those directions feel right for you?"

This conversation helps David recognize that his authentic interests can integrate with his academic strengths rather than competing with them.

Supporting Major Life Decisions

Transition planning involves decisions that feel enormous to teenagers because they lack experience with major life choices. MI principles help teens approach these decisions thoughtfully without becoming paralyzed by their magnitude:

Decision-Making Process Support

Break Down Big Decisions: Help teens understand that major life decisions are actually series of smaller decisions that can be made gradually.

Example: "Choosing a career doesn't have to happen all at once. You can choose a college program that keeps multiple options open, then make more specific career decisions as you learn more about yourself and different fields."

Explore Decision-Making Values: Help teens identify what makes a good decision for them personally.

Questions:

- "What would make you feel confident about a major decision?"

- "How do you want to balance different factors like family input, practical considerations, and personal interests?"

- "What role do you want others to play in your decision-making process?"

Address Decision Anxiety: Normalize anxiety about major decisions and help teens develop skills for managing uncertainty.

Reflection: "It makes sense that these decisions feel overwhelming – you're making choices about things you haven't experienced yet, and everyone has opinions about what you should do."

Question: "What would help you feel more confident about navigating uncertainty?"

Working with Family Expectations

Many teens struggle with tension between their own emerging interests and family expectations or pressures. MI can help teens navigate these complex dynamics:

Explore Family Values: Help teens understand the values and concerns underlying family expectations.

Question: "What do you think your parents most want for you? What are they hoping these career choices will provide?"

Follow-up: "How do you feel about those hopes and concerns? Which ones resonate with your own values?"

Identify Common Ground: Help teens find areas where their interests align with family values.

Example: "It sounds like both you and your parents value financial security and meaningful work. You might have different ideas about what careers provide those things, but you share some core values."

Develop Communication Strategies: Support teens in having authentic conversations with families about their interests and concerns.

Question: "What would need to happen for you to feel comfortable sharing your real interests with your family?"

Follow-up: "How could you help them understand your perspective while also showing that you've heard their concerns?"

Managing Social Pressures

Peer relationships and social expectations significantly influence teen transition planning. Rather than dismissing these influences, MI helps teens integrate social considerations thoughtfully:

Acknowledge Social Influences: Recognize that social considerations are legitimate factors in teen decision-making.

Reflection: "It sounds like maintaining friendships is important to you as you think about college choices. That's actually a really normal and healthy consideration."

Explore Social Values: Help teens distinguish between social pressure and their own social values.

Questions:

- "What kinds of social connections are most important to you?"

- "How do you want your friendships to influence your major life decisions?"

- "What would it look like to make choices that honor your relationships without compromising your own goals?"

Develop Independence Within Relationships: Support teens in making autonomous decisions while maintaining valued relationships.

Question: "How could you make choices that feel right for you while still being a good friend to people you care about?"

Exploring Options Without Pressure

One of the biggest challenges in transition planning is helping teens explore options thoroughly without creating pressure to commit prematurely:

The Exploration vs. Commitment Balance

Permission for Uncertainty: Explicitly normalize not knowing what you want to do with your life at 17 or 18.

Statement: "Not knowing what you want to do for a career at your age is completely normal. Your job right now is exploring possibilities, not making final decisions."

Reversible vs. Irreversible Decisions: Help teens distinguish between decisions that can be changed and those with long-term consequences.

Example: "Choosing a college major feels permanent, but most people change majors at least once. Choosing whether to go to college at all is a bigger decision, but even that isn't necessarily permanent."

Low-Stakes Exploration: Encourage exploration activities that provide information without requiring commitment.

Suggestions:

- Job shadowing or informational interviews
- College visits or virtual tours
- Community college classes in areas of interest
- Volunteer work in potential career fields
- Internships or part-time jobs

Supporting Authentic Interest Development

Many teens struggle to identify their "real" interests because they've been focused on external expectations for so long. MI can help teens reconnect with their authentic curiosity:

Childhood Interest Exploration: Help teens remember what they loved doing before academic and social pressures became dominant.

Questions:

- "What did you love doing as a kid before you started worrying about whether you were good at it?"
- "If you had a free Saturday with no obligations, what would you choose to do?"
- "What topics do you find yourself researching online just because you're curious?"

Present Moment Awareness: Help teens notice their current experiences of engagement and interest.

Questions:

- "When do you feel most like yourself?"
- "What activities make you lose track of time?"
- "What kinds of conversations energize you rather than drain you?"

Value-Based Interest Development: Help teens connect their interests to their deeper values and aspirations.

Questions:

- "What problems in the world do you wish someone would solve?"

- "If you could make one thing better in your community, what would it be?"

- "What kind of impact do you want to have on other people's lives?"

Building Confidence for Next Steps

Transition planning isn't just about making decisions – it's about developing the confidence and skills to navigate future transitions throughout life:

Developing Decision-Making Skills

Teach Decision-Making Process: Help teens develop systematic approaches to making major decisions that they can use throughout life.

Process Example:

1. **Clarify the decision**: What exactly needs to be decided, and by when?

2. **Identify values and priorities**: What matters most in this decision?

3. **Generate options**: What are all the possible choices, including creative alternatives?

4. **Gather information**: What do you need to know to make an informed decision?

5. **Consider consequences**: What are the likely outcomes of different choices?

6. **Make a decision**: Choose based on your values and the information available.

7. **Evaluate and adjust**: How can you assess whether the decision is working and make adjustments if needed?

Practice with Smaller Decisions: Help teens apply decision-making skills to lower-stakes choices to build confidence.

Examples: Choosing classes, summer activities, part-time jobs, or volunteer opportunities.

Building Self-Advocacy Skills

Identify Personal Needs: Help teens understand what conditions help them thrive.

Questions:

- "What kinds of environments help you do your best work?"

- "What support do you need when you're learning something challenging?"

- "How do you prefer to receive feedback and guidance?"

Communication Skills Development

Practice Asking for Help: Many teens struggle to seek support when they need it. Transition planning provides opportunities to develop these crucial skills.

Questions:

- "Who could you talk to about your questions regarding different college programs?"

- "What would make it easier for you to ask for guidance when you need it?"

- "How do you prefer to receive advice and feedback from adults?"

Articulate Personal Goals: Help teens develop skills for communicating their interests and goals to others.

Practice: "How would you explain to a college admissions counselor what you're hoping to get out of your college experience?"

Follow-up: "How would you share your career interests with a potential employer during an interview?"

Resilience Building for Uncertainty

Normalize Course Corrections: Help teens understand that changing directions is normal and often beneficial rather than a sign of failure.

Example: "Most successful adults have changed career paths multiple times. The skills you develop in one area often transfer to others in unexpected ways."

Develop Growth Mindset: Support teens in viewing challenges and setbacks as learning opportunities rather than evidence of inadequacy.

Reflection: "When you think about trying something new and potentially struggling with it, how do you want to handle those challenges?"

Question: "What would help you maintain confidence when you encounter difficulties in college or career exploration?"

Build Support Network Awareness: Help teens identify and cultivate relationships that will support them through future transitions.

Questions:

- "Who in your life helps you think through difficult decisions?"

- "What kinds of support are most helpful to you when you're facing uncertainty?"

- "How do you want to maintain connections with people who matter to you as you transition to the next phase of life?"

Practical Transition Planning Strategies

The Values-First College Search

Instead of starting with college rankings or parental preferences, begin with student values and work outward:

Step 1: Values Clarification *Exercise*: Have students identify their top 5 values from a comprehensive list, then discuss how these values might influence their college experience preferences.

Step 2: Environment Preferences *Questions*:

- "What size community helps you thrive?"

- "How important is geographic location to your well-being?"

- "What role do you want extracurricular activities to play in your college experience?"

Step 3: Academic Interest Integration *Approach*: Rather than choosing colleges based on specific majors, identify colleges that support exploration in areas of interest while maintaining flexibility.

Step 4: Practical Considerations *Discussion*: Address financial constraints, family expectations, and logistical considerations after establishing personal preferences.

The Skills-Based Career Exploration

Help teens identify transferable skills they enjoy using rather than focusing solely on specific career titles:

Skill Identification Process: *Question*: "What activities make you feel competent and engaged? What skills are you using during those times?"

Examples: Problem-solving, creative expression, helping others, organizing information, working with your hands, communicating ideas, analyzing data.

Skill Application Exploration: *Question*: "How might these skills be used in different career contexts? What industries or roles would value these abilities?"

Experience Seeking: *Approach*: Encourage teens to seek experiences that allow them to use preferred skills in different contexts rather than job shadowing specific careers.

The Gap Year Consideration

For students unsure about immediate college enrollment, explore gap year possibilities using MI principles:

Explore Motivations: *Questions*:

- "What appeals to you about taking time between high school and college?"

- "What concerns do you have about starting college immediately?"

- "What would you want to accomplish during a gap year?"

Address Family Concerns: *Approach*: Help teens understand family concerns about gap years while advocating for their own needs.

Questions:

- "What do you think your family is worried about regarding a gap year?"

- "How could you address their concerns while still considering this option?"

Structured Planning: *Support*: If gap year interests persist, help teens develop structured plans that address growth, experience, and preparation for future education.

Case Study: Supporting Non-Traditional Paths

Alex's Community College Choice:

Alex is a capable student whose friends are all applying to four-year colleges, but they're interested in studying automotive technology at the community college. They're worried about disappointing their academic-focused family and being judged by peers.

MI-Informed Support Process:

Counselor: "Alex, help me understand what draws you to automotive technology. What's your experience been with that kind of work?"

Alex: "I love working on cars. I've been helping my uncle in his shop since I was little, and I'm good at diagnosing problems and figuring out solutions. It just feels right to me."

Counselor: "It sounds like you've discovered something you're both passionate about and skilled at. That's actually pretty rare and valuable. What concerns do you have about pursuing that interest?"

Alex: "My parents always assumed I'd go to a four-year college because I have good grades. They think community college is settling for less. And my friends keep asking why I want to be 'just a mechanic.'"

Counselor: "So you're feeling pressure from people who see different educational paths as having different values. What's your own perspective on the value of automotive technology work?"

Alex: "I think it's really important work. People depend on their vehicles, and skilled technicians are always needed. Plus, the technology is getting so advanced – hybrid systems, computer diagnostics, electric vehicles. It's actually pretty high-tech now."

Counselor: "You see automotive technology as both personally fulfilling and socially valuable, and you recognize that it involves sophisticated technical skills. How do you think about balancing your own interests with other people's expectations?"

Alex: "I want my family to be proud of me, but I also want to do work that feels meaningful to me. Maybe there's a way to do both?"

Counselor: "What would it look like to pursue automotive technology in a way that honors both your interests and your family's hopes for your education?"

Alex: "Well, I could start at community college and then maybe transfer to a four-year program in automotive engineering. Or I could get certified as a technician and then eventually open my own shop."

Counselor: "Those sound like paths that combine your hands-on interests with longer-term educational and business goals. How could you share this kind of thinking with your family?"

This conversation helps Alex develop confidence in their interests while finding ways to address family concerns and social pressures.

Long-Term Perspective on Transition Planning

Effective transition planning recognizes that the decisions teens make at 17 or 18 are not permanent life sentences but rather first steps in ongoing development:

Developmental Appropriateness

Phase-Appropriate Expectations: Recognize that teens are choosing initial directions, not final destinations.

Message: "The goal isn't to choose the perfect career at 18. The goal is to choose next steps that keep you moving toward the kind of person you want to become."

Skill Development Focus: Emphasize that college and early career experiences are opportunities to develop capacities that will serve them throughout life.

Examples: Critical thinking, communication, problem-solving, collaboration, cultural competence, adaptability.

Identity Integration: Support teens in making choices that align with their emerging sense of self while remaining open to continued growth and change.

Preparing for Lifelong Transitions

Transition Skills: Help teens develop skills for navigating future life transitions, not just the current one.

Skills: Self-reflection, information gathering, decision-making, communication, adaptation, resilience.

Support Network Development: Encourage teens to build relationships and support systems that will help them through future challenges and changes.

Self-Knowledge: Support teens in developing ongoing awareness of their values, strengths, interests, and growth areas.

What This Means for the Future

The transition planning work you do with teenagers creates foundations that extend far beyond college and career choices. When teens learn to make decisions based on their authentic interests and values, when they develop skills for navigating uncertainty, and when they build confidence in their ability to handle whatever comes next, they're prepared not just for their next step but for a lifetime of thoughtful choices.

The MI principles that guide transition planning – collaboration over control, curiosity about the teen's perspective, respect for their autonomy, and faith in their capacity for growth – these same principles that support teens through the practical applications we've explored throughout this book now prepare both teens and adults for the hands-on work of change.

Part IV: Teen Worksheets

Chapter 12: Values Exploration

Seventeen-year-old Mia sits in her bedroom staring at a college application essay prompt: "Describe your core values and how they will influence your college experience." She's been staring at the blank screen for an hour. Her first draft started with "I value hard work and success," but that felt hollow and generic. Her second attempt focused on helping others, but she couldn't think of specific examples that felt authentic.

Frustrated, she texts her older sister: "How do I figure out what I actually value? Like, really value, not what I think I'm supposed to say."

Her sister's response surprises her: "Think about the last time you got really angry about something. What value was being violated?"

Suddenly, Mia has a starting point. Last month, she got furious when she saw classmates excluding a new student from their lunch table. Not just annoyed – genuinely angry. And when her part-time job required her to throw away perfectly good food instead of donating it to food banks, she felt physically sick about the waste.

For the first time, Mia begins to see her actual values emerging: fairness, inclusion, and stewardship of resources. These aren't the values she thought she should have – they're the values that actually drive her emotional responses and choices.

This moment illustrates why values exploration is so crucial for teenagers. **Values aren't abstract concepts to be learned – they're internal compass points that already exist within teens, waiting to be recognized and named.** But in a world full of external expectations, social media comparisons, and pressure to present the "right" image, many teens lose touch with their authentic values.

The exercises in this chapter help teens reconnect with what matters most to them personally, not what they think should matter or what others expect them to value.

Understanding Teen Values Development

Values formation during adolescence follows predictable patterns that inform how we approach values exploration:

Values vs. Beliefs: Values are fundamental principles that guide behavior and decision-making, while beliefs are specific ideas about how the world works. Values tend to be more stable and personal, while beliefs can change with new information (Rokeach, 1973).

Example:

- Value: Justice and fairness
- Belief: The best way to achieve justice is through specific legal reforms

Values vs. Goals: Values are ongoing principles that guide multiple goals over time, while goals are specific outcomes teens want to achieve. Values provide the "why" behind goals (Deci & Ryan, 2000).

Example:

- Value: Creative expression
- Goals: Join the drama club, learn guitar, major in art

Values vs. Interests: Interests are activities or topics that capture attention, while values are the underlying principles that make certain interests meaningful. Understanding this distinction helps teens see connections between different interests that share common values.

Example:

- Value: Understanding how things work

- Interests: Science experiments, taking apart electronics, coding, mystery novels

Developmental Considerations for Values Exploration

Identity Formation Integration: Values exploration during adolescence happens alongside identity formation. Teens aren't just discovering what they value – they're deciding who they want to be (Arnett, 2000).

Social Context Influence: Peer relationships and social groups heavily influence which values teens feel comfortable expressing, even if those values don't reflect their authentic priorities.

Family Values Integration: Teens must navigate the relationship between family values they've absorbed and their own emerging value system. This often involves integration rather than rejection.

Abstract Thinking Development: As teens develop capacity for abstract thinking, they can engage with values in more sophisticated ways, but they still need concrete connections to their lived experience.

What Matters Most Exercises

These exercises help teens identify their core values through reflection on their actual experiences, emotions, and choices rather than abstract concepts.

The Peak Experience Values Discovery

Purpose: Help teens identify values by exploring moments when they felt most alive, engaged, and authentic.

Instructions:

1. **Identify Peak Experiences**: "Think of 2-3 times in your life when you felt most engaged, energized, and like you were being your best self. These don't have to be major achievements – they could be everyday moments that felt particularly meaningful."

2. **Detailed Exploration**: For each experience, explore:

   o   What were you doing?

   o   Who were you with?

   o   What made this moment feel special?

   o   What values were you expressing through your actions?

3. **Pattern Recognition**: "Looking across these experiences, what values show up repeatedly? What principles were guiding your behavior during these meaningful moments?"

Example Process with Alex:

Alex's Peak Experience: "Last summer I volunteered at a day camp for kids with disabilities. There was this one kid, Jamie, who was really shy and wouldn't participate in activities. I spent extra time with him, and by the end of the week he was laughing and playing with other kids."

Values Exploration:

- "What made this experience meaningful to you?"

- "I felt like I made a real difference in Jamie's life. And I got to see him discover confidence he didn't know he had."

- "What values were you expressing through your actions with Jamie?"

- "I guess... patience, believing in people's potential, not giving up on someone just because they're different."

- "How do those values show up in other areas of your life?"

The Anger Values Assessment

Purpose: Use emotional responses to identify violated values, since anger often signals that something we care about has been threatened or violated.

Instructions:

1. **Identify Anger Triggers**: "Think about times in the past year when you felt genuinely angry or frustrated – not just annoyed, but really upset about something."

2. **Values Behind the Anger**: For each situation, explore:

   o   What exactly made you angry?

   o   What principle or value was being violated?

   o   What would have needed to happen for you to feel the situation was fair or right?

3. **Pattern Recognition**: "Looking across these situations, what values were being threatened? What do these anger responses tell you about what you care about?"

Example Process with Sofia:

Sofia's Anger Experience: "I got really mad when our group project grade was based only on the final presentation, not on who actually did the work. Two people in our group did nothing, but they got the same grade as those of us who worked hard."

Values Exploration:

- "What specifically made you angry about this situation?"

- "It wasn't fair. People who didn't contribute got rewarded the same as people who worked hard."

- "What value was being violated?"

- "Fairness, I guess. And... recognizing effort. I value hard work being acknowledged."

- "How does this value show up in other areas of your life?"

The Role Model Values Analysis

Purpose: Help teens identify values by exploring what they admire in others, since admiration often reflects our own value system.

Instructions:

1. **Identify Role Models**: "Think of 2-3 people you really admire – they could be people you know personally, public figures, fictional characters, or historical figures."

2. **Admiration Analysis**: For each person, explore:

   o What specifically do you admire about this person?

   o What qualities or actions make them inspiring to you?

   o What values do they represent or express?

3. **Personal Connection**: "How do these values connect to your own life? Which of these values do you want to express more fully in your own choices?"

Example Process with Jordan:

Jordan's Role Model: "I really admire my older cousin Maya. She's studying environmental engineering and works part-time at a community garden."

Values Exploration:

- "What specifically do you admire about Maya?"

- "She's doing work that she cares about, not just what pays well. And she's trying to solve real problems that affect people."

- "What values does Maya represent for you?"

- "Using your skills for something meaningful, caring about the environment, not just focusing on money but on making things better."

- "How do those values connect to choices you want to make in your own life?"

The Decision Values Archaeology

Purpose: Help teens recognize their values by examining past decisions, since our choices often reflect our priorities even when we're not conscious of them.

Instructions:

1. **Identify Significant Decisions**: "Think of 2-3 decisions you've made in the past year – they could be about classes, activities, relationships, or how you spend your time."

2. **Decision Archaeology**: For each decision, explore:

   - What factors influenced your choice?

   - What were you hoping to achieve or avoid?

   - Looking back, what values guided your decision?

3. **Pattern Recognition**: "Across these decisions, what values seem to consistently influence your choices?"

Interactive Values Card Sorts

Values card sorts provide structured ways for teens to prioritize their values and explore relationships between different values.

The Basic Values Card Sort

Materials: Create cards with 50-60 values that resonate with teenagers. Include a mix of traditional values and contemporary concerns.

Sample Values for Teen Card Sort:

- Authenticity
- Adventure
- Creativity
- Justice
- Independence
- Connection
- Excellence
- Fun
- Security
- Growth
- Recognition
- Service
- Beauty
- Challenge

155

- Spirituality

- Innovation

- Tradition

- Freedom

- Balance

- Impact

Process:

1. **Initial Sort**: Have teens sort values into three piles:

    o Very Important to Me

    o Somewhat Important to Me

    o Not Important to Me

2. **Top Values Selection**: From the "Very Important" pile, ask teens to select their top 10 values.

3. **Priority Ranking**: From those 10, select the top 5 most important values.

4. **Final Prioritization**: From those 5, identify the top 3 core values.

5. **Reflection Discussion**:

    o Were any of your final values surprising?

    o How do these values show up in your current life?

    o Where might you want to express these values more fully?

The Values Conflict Sort

Purpose: Help teens explore what happens when values conflict and how to navigate competing priorities.

Process:

1. **Scenario Presentation**: Present teens with realistic scenarios where values might conflict.

Example Scenario: "You have the opportunity to take a prestigious internship that would look great on college applications, but it would require you to miss your best friend's important family event and would involve working for a company whose practices you question."

2. **Values Identification**: "What values are at stake in this situation?"

- Achievement/Success
- Loyalty/Friendship
- Authenticity/Integrity
- Family/Relationships

3. **Priority Exploration**: "When these values conflict, how do you decide which ones take priority?"

4. **Integration Seeking**: "Are there ways to honor multiple values, even if you can't fully satisfy all of them?"

The Life Areas Values Mapping

Purpose: Help teens see how their core values might be expressed differently across various life areas.

Process:

1. **Life Areas Identification**: Ask teens to identify the major areas of their current life:

- School/Academics

- Family Relationships

- Friendships

- Romantic Relationships

- Work/Employment

- Extracurricular Activities

- Personal Time

- Future Planning

2. **Values Mapping**: For each life area, explore:

   - Which of your core values are you expressing well in this area?

   - Which values do you want to express more fully?

   - What would it look like to align this area more closely with your values?

3. **Integration Planning**: "Looking across all life areas, where do you see the biggest gaps between your values and your current choices?"

Connecting Values to Daily Choices

The most important aspect of values exploration is helping teens see how their identified values can guide everyday decisions and choices.

The Values-Behavior Gap Analysis

Purpose: Help teens recognize where their daily choices align with their stated values and where gaps exist.

Process:

1. **Time Audit**: Have teens track how they spend their time for a week, noting major time commitments and daily choices.

2. **Values Alignment Assessment**: For each major time commitment, ask:

   o Which of my core values does this activity express?

   o Where am I spending time on things that don't reflect my values?

   o What values am I not expressing through how I spend my time?

3. **Gap Identification**: "Where do you see the biggest differences between what you say you value and how you actually spend your time and energy?"

4. **Small Step Planning**: "What small changes could you make to better align your daily choices with your values?"

The Decision-Making Values Filter

Purpose: Teach teens to use their values as a decision-making tool for both small and large choices.

The Values Filter Process:

1. **Clarify the Decision**: What exactly needs to be decided?

2. **Identify Options**: What are all the possible choices?

3. **Values Check**: For each option, ask:

   o Which of my core values would this choice express?

   o Which values might this choice compromise?

   o How well does this option align with what matters most to me?

4. **Integration Seeking**: Is there a choice that honors multiple values, or do I need to prioritize?

5. **Decision and Reflection**: After choosing, reflect on how the decision feels in relation to your values.

Example: Choosing Between Activities

Marcus's Decision: Whether to join the debate team or get a part-time job.

Values Filter Application:

- Core Values: Learning, Financial Independence, Excellence

- Debate Team: Strong alignment with learning and excellence values, no alignment with financial independence

- Part-time Job: Strong alignment with financial independence, potential alignment with learning (life skills), uncertain alignment with excellence

- Integration Seeking: Is there a way to do both part-time, or choose one now and the other later?

- Decision Factors: Which values are most important right now given his current situation and future goals?

Values-Based Goal Setting

Purpose: Help teens set goals that reflect their authentic values rather than external expectations.

Process:

1. **Values Foundation**: Start with teens' identified core values rather than predetermined goal categories.

2. **Values Expression Exploration**: For each core value, ask:

- How do you want to express this value more fully in your life?

- What would it look like if this value guided more of your choices?

- What specific changes would reflect this value?

3. **Goal Development**: Transform values expressions into specific, actionable goals.

4. **Values Alignment Check**: For each goal, confirm:

- Does this goal reflect my authentic values or external expectations?

- Will achieving this goal help me become the person I want to be?

Example: Values-Based Goal Setting

Emma's Core Value: Creative expression and authenticity

Values Expression Exploration:

- "I want to express my creativity through writing and art"

- "I want to share my authentic perspective rather than just saying what I think people want to hear"

- "I want to find ways to use creativity to connect with others"

Resulting Goals:

- Start a creative writing club at school

- Submit writing to the school literary magazine

- Create art pieces that reflect my actual interests rather than what gets good grades

- Find opportunities to collaborate creatively with friends

Teen-Friendly Values Assessment Tools

Traditional values assessments are often designed for adults and may not capture the developmental concerns and life contexts relevant to teenagers.

The Social Media Values Reflection

Purpose: Use teens' social media behavior to explore their values, since social media choices often reflect what people want to be associated with.

Instructions:

1. **Social Media Audit**: Have teens look at their recent social media posts, likes, shares, and follows.

2. **Values Reflection Questions**:

   o What values are reflected in the content you choose to share?

   o What causes or issues do you engage with online?

   o What kind of image are you presenting, and how does that connect to your values?

   o Where do you see gaps between your online presence and your actual values?

3. **Alignment Planning**: "How could you use social media in ways that better reflect your authentic values?"

The Future Self Values Interview

Purpose: Help teens explore their values by imagining their future selves and working backwards to identify what values would need to guide their choices.

Instructions:

1. **Future Self Visualization**: "Imagine yourself 10 years from now, living a life that feels meaningful and authentic to you. Don't worry about being realistic – focus on what would feel fulfilling."

2. **Future Self Interview**: Ask your future self:

   o   What does your typical day look like?

   o   What work are you doing, and why is it meaningful to you?

   o   What relationships are important in your life?

   o   What are you most proud of having accomplished?

   o   What challenges have you overcome?

3. **Values Identification**: "What values would your future self need to have lived by to create this kind of life?"

4. **Present Connection**: "Which of those values are you already expressing? Which ones do you want to start expressing more fully now?"

The Values and Identity Integration Assessment

Purpose: Help teens explore how their values connect to their developing sense of identity.

Process:

1. **Identity Aspects Identification**: Have teens identify different aspects of their identity:

   o   Cultural/ethnic identity

   o   Gender identity

   o   Academic identity

- o Social identity

- o Creative identity

- o Athletic identity

- o Family role identity

2. **Values Connection Exploration**: For each identity aspect, explore:

   - o What values are important within this aspect of your identity?

   - o Where do you see conflicts between different identity-related values?

   - o Which identity aspects feel most authentic to who you want to become?

3. **Integration Planning**: "How can you honor multiple aspects of your identity while staying true to your core values?"

Case Study: Complete Values Exploration Process

Working with Jasmine:

Jasmine is a 16-year-old who feels confused about her direction and pressured by others' expectations. Here's how a complete values exploration process might unfold:

Step 1: Peak Experience Discovery *Facilitator*: "Tell me about a time recently when you felt most like yourself – most engaged and energized."

Jasmine: "Last month I organized a fundraiser at school for the animal shelter. I got different clubs to participate, designed flyers, coordinated with the shelter staff. It was stressful but really satisfying."

Values Identification: Helping others, organization, bringing people together, animal welfare

Step 2: Anger Values Assessment *Facilitator*: "What's something that really bothers you or makes you angry?"

Jasmine: "When people are mean to animals, or when people say they care about something but don't actually do anything about it. Like, don't just post about environmental issues – actually change your behavior."

Values Identification: Compassion, authenticity, taking action on beliefs

Step 3: Role Model Analysis *Facilitator*: "Who do you really admire?"

Jasmine: "Jane Goodall and my aunt who's a veterinarian. They both dedicated their lives to helping animals and they didn't let people tell them it wasn't practical."

Values Identification: Following your passion, perseverance, service to something larger than yourself

Step 4: Values Integration *Core Values Identified*: Compassion, authenticity, service, bringing people together, following your passion

Step 5: Current Life Alignment *Gaps Identified*: Jasmine realizes she's been focusing on academics that lead to "practical" careers but not exploring her genuine interest in animal welfare and environmental issues.

Step 6: Values-Based Planning *Changes*: Join environmental club, volunteer at animal shelter, explore colleges with strong environmental science programs, have honest conversation with parents about her interests.

Making Values Stick

Values exploration is just the beginning. The real work involves helping teens integrate their identified values into their daily decision-making and long-term planning.

Regular Values Check-Ins

Monthly Values Reflection:

- How have I expressed my core values this month?

- Where have I made choices that didn't align with my values?

- What do I want to do differently going forward?

Decision-Making Values Application:

- Before making significant choices, ask: "How do my options align with my core values?"

- After making decisions, reflect: "How did my values influence this choice?"

Values Communication Skills

Articulating Values to Others: Help teens develop skills for communicating their values to parents, friends, and other important people:

- "This is important to me because..."

- "Based on what I value, I think..."

- "I want to make choices that reflect my belief in..."

Values-Based Boundary Setting: Support teens in setting boundaries that protect their values:

- "I'm not comfortable with that because it conflicts with my values around..."

- "I need to make choices that align with what's important to me, which is..."

Values and Identity Development

Identity Integration: Help teens see how their values connect to their developing sense of self and their future aspirations.

Values Consistency: Support teens in developing consistency between their stated values and their actual choices, while allowing for growth and change.

Values Flexibility: Help teens understand that values can be expressed differently in different contexts while maintaining their core importance.

What Values Exploration Builds Toward

Values exploration creates the foundation for all other change work with teenagers. When teens have clarity about what matters most to them, they can use that clarity to evaluate options, make decisions, and stay motivated during challenging periods.

The values work you do with teens becomes the foundation for change planning, goal setting, and decision-making. It provides the "why" that sustains motivation when the "how" becomes difficult.

Moving Forward with Clear Direction

Once teens have identified their core values, they need tools for evaluating their readiness and motivation for specific changes. The scaling and measurement tools in the next section help teens assess where they are currently and how ready they feel to make changes that align with their values.

Values provide the destination – change rulers help teens figure out the route and timing for getting there.

Chapter 13: Change Rulers

Sixteen-year-old Carlos sits with his school counselor, having just identified that he values academic achievement, family respect, and personal growth. But he's struggling in his advanced math class and considering dropping down to the regular level. The conversation has been going in circles for twenty minutes.

"I know I should stick with advanced math because it's better for college," Carlos says. "But I'm getting C's and D's, and it's making me feel terrible about myself. Maybe I should drop down, but then I'd feel like I'm giving up."

His counselor tries a different approach: "Carlos, on a scale from 1 to 10, where 10 means staying in advanced math is extremely important to you personally, and 1 means it's not important at all, where would you put yourself?"

Carlos thinks for a moment. "Maybe a 7? It is important to me."

"And on the same scale, where 10 means you're completely confident you can succeed in advanced math with the right support, and 1 means you have no confidence at all, where are you?"

"That's harder... maybe a 4?"

Suddenly, the issue becomes clear. Carlos values staying in the advanced class (importance = 7), but he lacks confidence in his ability to succeed (confidence = 4). The solution isn't about whether he should or shouldn't stay in the class – it's about building his confidence through better support, study strategies, or tutoring.

This simple scaling exercise transforms a circular conversation into focused action planning. **Change rulers provide visual, intuitive**

ways for teens to assess their motivation and readiness for different changes. Instead of getting stuck in abstract discussions about what teens "should" do, rulers help them evaluate where they are and what needs to shift for change to become more likely.

Understanding the Psychology of Change Measurement

Scaling tools work particularly well with adolescents because they match how the teenage brain naturally processes information:

Visual Processing Preference: Teens often think more visually than verbally. Rulers provide concrete visual representations of abstract concepts like motivation and confidence (Blakemore, 2018).

Comparative Thinking: Adolescent cognitive development involves increasingly sophisticated ability to make comparisons. Scaling tools capitalize on this natural tendency.

Autonomy Support: Rulers allow teens to self-assess rather than having adults assess for them, supporting their developmental need for autonomy.

Concrete Abstract Bridge: Scaling tools help bridge the gap between abstract concepts (like "readiness for change") and concrete thinking that teens can more easily access.

Emotional Regulation Support: Visual scales help teens step back from intense emotions and gain perspective on their experiences.

Visual Scaling Tools

The power of scaling tools lies in their simplicity and immediate visual impact. Here are the essential scaling tools for motivational work with teens:

The Basic Change Ruler

Purpose: Help teens assess their overall readiness for a specific change on a simple 1-10 scale.

Instructions: "On a scale from 1 to 10, where 1 means you're not at all ready to make this change, and 10 means you're completely ready to make this change right now, where would you put yourself?"

Follow-up Questions:

- "What makes you a [number they chose] instead of a 1?"

- "What would need to happen for you to move up one number?"

- "Have you been at different numbers on this scale at different times?"

Visual Enhancement: Create actual ruler graphics or use a simple line with numbers 1-10 marked. Have teens point to or mark their position.

The Motivation vs. Ability Ruler

Purpose: Help teens distinguish between wanting to change and feeling capable of change.

Two-Scale Assessment:

Scale 1 - Importance/Motivation: "On a scale from 1 to 10, how important is this change to you personally?"

Scale 2 - Confidence/Ability: "On a scale from 1 to 10, how confident are you that you could make this change if you decided to?"

Interpretation Guide:

- High Importance + High Confidence = Ready for action

- High Importance + Low Confidence = Need skill building, support, or different approach

- Low Importance + High Confidence = Need motivation building or values clarification

- Low Importance + Low Confidence = Premature for change focus; need exploration

Example with Maya's Exercise Goals:

Maya wants to exercise regularly but keeps skipping her planned workouts.

Importance Scale: "How important is regular exercise to you personally?" *Maya*: "8 – I really want to be healthier and have more energy."

Confidence Scale: "How confident are you that you can exercise regularly?" *Maya*: "3 – I keep planning to work out but I never follow through."

Interpretation: Maya is motivated (8) but lacks confidence (3). The focus should be on building her confidence through smaller goals, better planning, or addressing obstacles rather than trying to increase her motivation.

The Competing Values Ruler

Purpose: Help teens visualize internal conflicts when different values compete.

Process:

1. **Identify Competing Values**: "What different things matter to you in this situation?"

2. **Create Competing Scales**: Set up scales for each competing value.

3. **Assess Each Value**: Rate the importance of each competing value in the current decision.

171

4. **Explore the Tension**: "How do you handle it when different things you care about seem to conflict?"

Example with David's Social vs. Academic Conflict:

David is torn between spending time with friends and studying for finals.

Social Connection Scale: "How important is spending time with friends right now?" *David*: "9 – I feel disconnected from everyone because I've been studying so much."

Academic Achievement Scale: "How important is doing well on finals?" *David*: "8 – These grades really matter for my college applications."

Values Integration Discussion: "Both social connection and academic achievement are really important to you. What would it look like to honor both values during finals week?"

Importance and Confidence Rulers

The distinction between importance (how much teens care about change) and confidence (how capable they feel of making change) is crucial for effective intervention planning.

The Importance Ruler Deep Exploration

Basic Question: "On a scale from 1-10, how important is [specific change] to you personally?"

Follow-up Exploration for Low Importance (1-4):

- "What would need to be different about this change for it to feel more important to you?"

- "Who else thinks this change is important? How do you feel about their opinions?"

- "What would make this change matter more to you personally?"

- "What values might this change connect to that we haven't explored yet?"

Follow-up Exploration for Moderate Importance (5-7):

- "What makes this change feel somewhat important to you?"

- "What holds you back from feeling like it's more important?"

- "What would push this up to an 8 or 9 for you?"

- "What concerns do you have about making this change a higher priority?"

Follow-up Exploration for High Importance (8-10):

- "This clearly matters a lot to you. What makes it so important?"

- "How does this change connect to your values and goals?"

- "What would happen if you didn't make this change?"

- "Given how important this is, what gets in the way of moving forward?"

The Confidence Ruler Deep Exploration

Basic Question: "On a scale from 1-10, how confident are you that you could make this change if you decided to?"

Follow-up Exploration for Low Confidence (1-4):

- "What makes this change feel difficult or impossible right now?"

- "What would need to be different for you to feel more confident?"

- "Have you ever made similar changes successfully? What helped then?"

- "Who could support you in making this change?"

- "What smaller step might you feel more confident about?"

Follow-up Exploration for Moderate Confidence (5-7):

- "What gives you some confidence about making this change?"

- "What concerns do you have about your ability to follow through?"

- "What resources or support would boost your confidence?"

- "What obstacles are you anticipating, and how might you handle them?"

Follow-up Exploration for High Confidence (8-10):

- "You feel pretty confident about this change. What gives you that confidence?"

- "What strengths or resources do you have that support this change?"

- "What would you do if you encountered unexpected obstacles?"

- "Given your high confidence, what would help you get started?"

Case Study: Using Importance and Confidence Rulers

Sophia's Screen Time Reduction Goal:

Sophia, 17, wants to reduce her social media use because she feels it's affecting her sleep and mood, but she keeps falling back into old patterns.

Importance Assessment: *Counselor*: "On a scale from 1-10, how important is reducing your screen time to you personally?"

Sophia: "7. It's pretty important because I can see it's affecting my sleep and I waste so much time scrolling."

Follow-up: "What makes it a 7 instead of a 9 or 10?"

Sophia: "Well, I also use social media to stay connected with friends, and I don't want to miss out on what's happening."

Confidence Assessment: *Counselor*: "On that same scale, how confident are you that you could reduce your screen time if you decided to?"

Sophia: "Maybe a 3. I've tried before and I always end up back where I started."

Follow-up: "What makes it hard to stick with screen time limits?"

Sophia: "I set these big goals like 'only 30 minutes a day' and then I feel like a failure when I go over. Plus, I'm bored without my phone and I don't know what else to do."

Intervention Planning: Based on moderate importance (7) and low confidence (3), the intervention should focus on:

- Building confidence through smaller, achievable goals
- Addressing the competing value of social connection
- Developing alternative activities for boredom
- Creating more realistic and flexible screen time goals

Progress Tracking Sheets

Visual progress tracking helps teens see change as a gradual process rather than an all-or-nothing outcome. This is especially important for adolescents who may have unrealistic expectations about how quickly change should happen.

The Weekly Rulers Check-In

Purpose: Track changes in importance and confidence over time to identify patterns and progress.

Format: Create a simple weekly tracking sheet with spaces for:

Week of: _____

Goal/Change I'm Working On: _____

This Week's Ratings:

- Importance (1-10): ___

- Confidence (1-10): ___

What Happened This Week:

- What went well: _____

- What was challenging: _____

- What I learned about myself: _____

Next Week's Focus:

- One thing I want to try: _____

- Support I need: _____

The Change Readiness Tracker

Purpose: Help teens track multiple dimensions of readiness across time.

Weekly Assessment Categories:

Motivation Level (1-10): How much do I want this change right now?

Energy Level (1-10): How much energy do I have for working on this change?

Support Level (1-10): How supported do I feel by others in making this change?

Stress Level (1-10): How stressed am I about other things that might interfere?

Success Feeling (1-10): How successful do I feel with this change so far?

Pattern Recognition Questions:

- What patterns do I notice in my ratings over time?

- What external factors seem to affect my readiness for change?

- When am I most/least ready to work on this change?

- What do these patterns tell me about how to approach this change?

The Obstacles and Supports Tracker

Purpose: Help teens identify what helps and what hinders their change efforts.

Weekly Tracking Format:

This Week's Supports (Things that helped me with my change goal):

- Internal supports (my thoughts, feelings, skills):

  _____

- External supports (people, resources, circumstances):

  _____

This Week's Obstacles (Things that made my change goal harder):

- Internal obstacles (my thoughts, feelings, habits):

  _____

- External obstacles (people, circumstances, barriers):

  _____

Learning Questions:

- Which supports can I cultivate more?

- Which obstacles can I address or work around?

- What patterns do I see in what helps vs. what hinders me?

Goal Visualization Exercises

Visual goal representation helps teens make abstract future outcomes more concrete and motivating.

The Future Self Visualization Ruler

Purpose: Help teens connect current change efforts to their future self and goals.

Process:

1. **Future Self Description**: "Describe yourself one year from now if you successfully make this change. What would be different about your life?"

2. **Values Alignment Scaling**: "On a scale from 1-10, how well would that future self be living according to your core values?"

3. **Current State Assessment**: "Where are you now on that same scale?"

4. **Gap Visualization**: "What would need to happen to move from where you are now to where you want to be?"

5. **Step-by-Step Scaling**: "What would each number on the scale from your current position to your goal look like in terms of concrete changes?"

The Change Journey Map

Purpose: Help teens visualize change as a journey with recognizable milestones rather than a single destination.

Process:

1. **Starting Point**: "Where are you now with this change?" (Mark on a visual journey map)

2. **Destination**: "Where do you want to end up?" (Mark endpoint on map)

3. **Milestone Identification**: "What would be the major milestones along this journey?" (Mark 3-5 points between start and finish)

4. **Current Progress**: "Where are you right now on this journey?"

5. **Next Milestone Focus**: "What's the next milestone you're working toward?"

6. **Pathway Planning**: "What's the path from where you are to the next milestone?"

The Motivation Meter Visualization

Purpose: Help teens understand that motivation naturally fluctuates and plan for different motivation levels.

Instructions:

1. **Create Motivation Meter**: Draw a meter with sections marked:

- Red Zone (1-3): Low motivation, high struggle

- Yellow Zone (4-6): Moderate motivation, some challenges

- Green Zone (7-10): High motivation, ready for action

2. **Current Position**: "Where is your motivation meter right now for this change?"

3. **Zone-Specific Planning**:

   - **Red Zone Strategies**: "What helps you get through low motivation times?"

   - **Yellow Zone Strategies**: "How can you build momentum when motivation is moderate?"

   - **Green Zone Strategies**: "How can you make the most of high motivation times?"

4. **Meter Movement Factors**: "What tends to move your meter up? What moves it down?"

Case Study: Complete Visualization Process

Working with Kevin on Academic Motivation:

Kevin, 16, is struggling with motivation for schoolwork and getting poor grades despite being capable.

Future Self Visualization: *Kevin's Future Self Description*: "I'm getting B's and A's, I feel proud of my work, and I'm not stressed about college applications because my grades are solid."

Values Alignment: "That future self would be at about an 8 for living my values of achievement and self-respect."

Current State: "I'm probably at a 3 right now."

Change Journey Mapping: *Starting Point*: "Failing most classes, feeling terrible about school" *Milestones*:

- Turning in assignments consistently

- Getting C's in most classes

- Getting B's in classes I care about

- Feeling proud of my academic effort *Destination*: "Strong student who feels confident about academics" *Current Position*: "Somewhere between starting point and first milestone"

Motivation Meter Assessment: *Current Motivation*: "4 - yellow zone. I want to do better but it feels overwhelming"

Zone-Specific Strategies:

- Red Zone: "Talk to counselor, focus on just one class"

- Yellow Zone: "Set small daily goals, celebrate small wins"

- Green Zone: "Tackle bigger projects, plan ahead for multiple classes"

Meter Movement Factors:

- Moves Up: "When I succeed at something, when teachers are encouraging"

- Moves Down: "When I fall behind, when I compare myself to other students"

Making Rulers Work for Different Types of Teens

For Perfectionistic Teens

Challenge: Perfectionistic teens may rate themselves harshly or expect to be at 10 immediately.

Adaptations:

- Normalize that 7s and 8s are excellent scores that indicate readiness for change

- Explore what "good enough" progress looks like

- Use rulers to show that change is gradual and imperfect

- Focus on progress rather than absolute numbers

Example: "You rated your confidence at 6, and you seem disappointed by that. What would it mean if 6 was actually a pretty good place to start from?"

For All-or-Nothing Teens

Challenge: Some teens see change as either complete success or total failure.

Adaptations:

- Use rulers to show that change happens in increments

- Celebrate movement between numbers, not just reaching 10

- Explore what different numbers actually look like in behavior

- Normalize fluctuation in ratings over time

Example: "You went from a 3 to a 5 in confidence this week. That's significant progress! What happened that moved you up two points?"

For Externally Motivated Teens

Challenge: Teens who are motivated primarily by others' expectations may have difficulty accessing their own importance ratings.

Adaptations:

- Spend extra time on values clarification before using rulers

- Ask about personal importance separate from others' expectations

- Explore what would make change important to them personally

- Use rulers to distinguish between their motivation and others' expectations

Example: "You rated importance at 8, but that seems to be based on what your parents want. What would your personal importance rating be?"

For Resistant or Ambivalent Teens

Challenge: Teens who are resistant to change may give low ratings across all scales.

Adaptations:

- Explore what makes ratings higher than 1 (finding existing motivation)

- Ask about worst-case scenarios if things don't change

- Use rulers to explore ambivalence rather than push for change

- Respect low ratings as valuable information rather than problems to solve

Example: "You rated importance at 2, which tells me this change doesn't feel personally meaningful to you right now. Help me understand what would need to be different for it to feel more important."

Advanced Ruler Techniques

The Relationship Ruler

Purpose: Help teens assess how changes might affect their relationships.

Process: "On a scale from 1-10, how much do you think [important person] would support you in making this change?"

Follow-up Questions:

- Who in your life would be most supportive of this change?

- Who might be least supportive?

- How important is others' support for you in making this change?

- What would help you get more support from people who matter to you?

The Cost-Benefit Ruler

Purpose: Help teens weigh the costs and benefits of change.

Process:

1. **Benefits Scale**: "On a scale from 1-10, how beneficial would this change be for you?"

2. **Costs Scale**: "On the same scale, how costly or difficult would this change be?"

3. **Cost-Benefit Analysis**: Explore the relationship between perceived benefits and costs.

Follow-up Questions:

- What would make the benefits feel more significant?

- What would reduce the costs or difficulty?

- How do you think about balancing short-term costs with long-term benefits?

The Timing Ruler

Purpose: Help teens assess whether now is the right time for specific changes.

Process: "On a scale from 1-10, where 10 means this is the perfect time to make this change and 1 means this is the worst possible time, where would you rate right now?"

Follow-up Questions:

- What makes this timing feel right/wrong for this change?

- What would need to be different for the timing to feel better?

- What other things are competing for your attention right now?

- How do you balance working on this change with other priorities?

Building Change Ruler Skills

Teaching Teens to Use Rulers Independently

Self-Assessment Skills:

- How to check in with themselves regularly about motivation and confidence

- When to use different types of rulers for different situations

- How to interpret their own ratings and plan accordingly

Decision-Making Integration:

- Using rulers to evaluate options before making choices

- Checking importance and confidence before committing to goals

- Using scaling to assess readiness for next steps

Communication Skills:

- How to share ruler assessments with parents, teachers, or other support people

- Using scales to explain their perspective on changes or goals

- Advocating for support based on their confidence assessments

What Rulers Reveal About Readiness

Change rulers provide crucial information that guides intervention approaches:

High Importance + High Confidence: Teen is ready for action planning and goal setting.

High Importance + Low Confidence: Focus on skill building, support, and breaking goals into smaller steps.

Low Importance + High Confidence: Work on motivation building and values clarification.

Low Importance + Low Confidence: Change may be premature; focus on exploration and relationship building.

Fluctuating Ratings: Normal part of change process; help teen understand and plan for motivation variations.

What This Builds Toward

Scaling tools provide the assessment foundation for effective change planning. Once teens understand where they are in terms of importance and confidence, they need decision-making tools that help them think through their options systematically.

The ruler work creates readiness for more sophisticated decision-making processes that account for the complex factors teens face in their actual lives – including social media influences, peer pressure, and future self considerations that traditional pros and cons approaches often miss.

Chapter 14: Pros and Cons 2.0

Eighteen-year-old Maya sits in her guidance counselor's office, staring at a traditional pros and cons list about taking a gap year before college. The "pros" column lists things like "travel opportunities" and "work experience." The "cons" column includes "delayed college start" and "potential loss of academic momentum."

But Maya feels frustrated. This list doesn't capture what she's really struggling with. She's worried about what her Instagram feed will look like when all her friends are posting college experiences while she's working at a local nonprofit. She's concerned about disappointing her parents, who immigrated to give her educational opportunities. She's wondering how this choice will affect her relationship with her boyfriend, who's planning to attend college in another state.

"This doesn't help," Maya tells her counselor. "It's like you're asking me to decide between 'adventure' and 'college success,' but that's not what I'm actually thinking about. I'm thinking about social media, family expectations, relationships, and what I'll regret when I'm older."

Maya's frustration illustrates why traditional decision-making tools often fail with teenagers. **Teens don't make decisions in abstract vacuums – they make decisions within complex social, emotional, and digital contexts that traditional pros and cons lists completely ignore.**

The decision-making tools in this chapter account for the realities of teenage life in the 21st century: social media influence, peer pressure, family dynamics, future self considerations, and the emotional complexity of choices that feel identity-defining.

Why Traditional Pros and Cons Don't Work for Teens

Standard pros and cons lists assume rational, individual decision-making that doesn't match how adolescent brains actually process choices:

Social Context Blindness: Traditional lists ignore the social implications of decisions, which are often the most important factors for teenagers whose brains are hyperresponsive to peer evaluation (Blakemore, 2018).

Emotional Minimization: Standard approaches treat emotions as separate from rational thinking, but teen decision-making is inherently emotional, and emotions provide important information about values and preferences.

Static Thinking: Traditional lists create snapshots of current thinking but don't account for how teens' perspectives and priorities change over time.

Individual Focus: Standard approaches assume individual decision-making, but teens make most important decisions within family systems and peer relationships that significantly influence outcomes.

Present-Moment Bias: Traditional lists often emphasize immediate pros and cons while minimizing future implications, which doesn't help teens develop long-term thinking skills.

Binary Framework: Pros vs. cons suggests that decisions are about choosing between good and bad options, rather than helping teens navigate complex decisions where multiple values compete.

Modern Decision-Making Aids

189

Contemporary decision-making tools for teens need to account for the digital, social, and emotionally complex world they actually inhabit.

The Values-Weighted Decision Matrix

Purpose: Help teens make decisions based on their personal values rather than just listing generic pros and cons.

Process:

1. **Identify the Decision**: Clearly state what needs to be decided.

2. **List Core Values**: Use the teen's previously identified core values (from Chapter 12) as decision criteria.

3. **Rate Each Option**: For each possible choice, rate how well it aligns with each core value (1-10 scale).

4. **Calculate Values Alignment**: See which option best supports the teen's authentic values overall.

Example: Maya's Gap Year Decision

Maya's Core Values: Personal growth, family respect, authentic relationships, financial responsibility, service to others

Option 1: Take Gap Year

- Personal growth: 9 (travel, work experience, life skills)

- Family respect: 4 (parents prefer immediate college)

- Authentic relationships: 6 (different path than friends, but honest to interests)

- Financial responsibility: 8 (earning money, avoiding student loans for a year)

- Service to others: 9 (working for nonprofit)

Option 2: Go Directly to College

- Personal growth: 6 (academic learning, some independence)

- Family respect: 9 (fulfilling parents' dreams)

- Authentic relationships: 7 (same path as friends)

- Financial responsibility: 5 (taking on debt immediately)

- Service to others: 5 (limited opportunities while studying)

Values Alignment Totals:

- Gap year: 36 points

- Direct to college: 32 points

Important Note: The numbers aren't the decision-maker – they're conversation starters. The real value comes from discussing why certain values score differently with different options.

The Multiple Perspectives Framework

Purpose: Help teens understand how different people in their lives might view their decision, and how much weight to give different perspectives.

Process:

1. **Identify Key Stakeholders**: Who has opinions about or will be affected by this decision?

2. **Perspective Taking**: For each stakeholder, consider:

   o How would they view each option?

   o What are they worried about?

   o What are they hoping for?

   o What values are driving their perspective?

3. **Influence Assessment**: How much weight do you want to give each person's perspective?

4. **Integration Planning**: How can you make a decision that honors important relationships while staying true to yourself?

Example: Maya's Stakeholder Analysis

Parents' Perspective:

- Preferred option: Direct to college

- Worries: Maya will lose academic momentum, miss opportunities

- Hopes: Maya will get education they couldn't, achieve financial security

- Values: Education, achievement, security

- Weight Maya wants to give: High (they're important to her and supporting her financially)

Best Friend's Perspective:

- Preferred option: Gap year sounds cool, but worried about drifting apart

- Worries: Different life experiences will change their friendship

- Hopes: Maya will be happy and they'll stay close

- Values: Friendship, shared experiences, authenticity

- Weight Maya wants to give: Medium (friendship matters, but friend will adjust)

Maya's Future Self Perspective:

- Preferred option: Unclear - depends on what she learns about herself

- Worries: Making the "wrong" choice, missing out on experiences

- Hopes: Making a choice that leads to authentic, meaningful life

- Values: Self-knowledge, no regrets, personal growth

- Weight Maya wants to give: Very high (she has to live with the consequences)

The Regret Minimization Framework

Purpose: Help teens think about long-term implications by considering what they might regret not trying.

Adapted from Jeff Bezos's decision-making framework, modified for teenage concerns:

Process:

1. **Future Self Visualization**: "Imagine yourself at age 30, looking back on this decision."

2. **Regret Assessment**: For each option, ask:

   - "What would 30-year-old you regret not trying?"

   - "What would 30-year-old you be glad you experienced?"

   - "What would 30-year-old you wish you had learned about yourself?"

3. **Learning Opportunity Evaluation**: Which option provides more opportunities to learn about yourself and what you want?

4. **Reversibility Assessment**: Which aspects of each choice can be changed later if needed?

Example: Maya's Regret Analysis

30-Year-Old Maya Looking Back on Gap Year:

- Might regret: Not having traditional college experience with friends

- Might be glad about: Taking time to figure out what she really wanted to study

- Would have learned: Whether she really likes nonprofit work, how to live independently

30-Year-Old Maya Looking Back on Direct College Entry:

- Might regret: Not taking time to explore interests before committing to expensive education

- Might be glad about: Starting career earlier, staying on traditional timeline

- Would have learned: Academic interests, how to succeed in structured environment

Maya's Reflection: "I think 30-year-old me would regret not taking the gap year more than not going to college immediately, because I can always go to college later, but this opportunity to work for the nonprofit and really think about what I want won't come again."

Digital-Age Decisional Balance Sheets

Modern teens need decision-making tools that account for digital and social media realities that didn't exist for previous generations.

The Social Media Reality Check

Purpose: Help teens honestly assess how social media considerations affect their decisions.

Process:

1. **Social Media Impact Assessment**: "How much is your decision influenced by how it will look on social media or what you'll be able to post about?"

2. **Online vs. Offline Reality Check**: "What will the online version of each choice look like vs. the actual daily reality?"

3. **FOMO Analysis**: "What are you afraid of missing out on with each option? How realistic are those fears?"

4. **Authentic vs. Performative Evaluation**: "Which choice feels more about living authentically vs. looking good to others online?"

Example: David's College Choice

David is choosing between a prestigious university and a smaller school with a better program in his area of interest.

Social Media Reality Check:

- Prestigious university: "Great for posts, impressive name-dropping, lots of 'likes' on acceptance announcement"

- Smaller school: "Less impressive posts, might have to explain why I chose it over more famous options"

Online vs. Offline Reality:

- Prestigious university: "Online looks amazing, but daily reality might be huge classes, intense competition, less personal attention"

- Smaller school: "Won't photograph as impressively, but daily reality includes small classes, professors who know my name, research opportunities"

David's Reflection: "I'm realizing I'm letting Instagram influence my college choice, which is pretty messed up. The smaller school actually fits better with what I want from college."

The Peer Pressure Decision Audit

Purpose: Help teens identify and evaluate peer influence on their decisions.

Process:

1. **Peer Influence Identification**: "How are your friends/peers influencing this decision?"

2. **Influence Type Assessment**: Is the influence:
   - Direct advice or pressure?
   - Modeling through their choices?
   - Unspoken expectations or norms?
   - Fear of being left out or judged?

3. **Peer Values vs. Personal Values**: "Are your friends' values about this decision similar to or different from your own values?"

4. **Long-term Relationship Considerations**: "How will each choice affect your relationships? How important is that to you?"

5. **Independence vs. Connection Balance**: "How do you want to balance making independent choices with maintaining important relationships?"

The Family Dynamics Decision Map

Purpose: Help teens navigate family expectations and dynamics in their decision-making.

Process:

1. **Family Values Identification**: "What values is your family expressing about this decision?"

2. **Spoken vs. Unspoken Expectations**: "What has your family directly said about what they want? What haven't they said directly but you know they're thinking?"

3. **Family History Consideration**: "How does your family's background or experiences influence their perspective on this decision?"

4. **Autonomy vs. Respect Balance**: "How do you want to balance making your own choice with respecting your family's input and support?"

5. **Communication Planning**: "How do you want to involve your family in your decision-making process?"

Example: Alex's Career Path Decision

Alex is torn between pursuing art (personal passion) and business (family expectation).

Family Values Analysis:

- Expressed values: Financial security, practical career choices, "stable" professions

- Family background: Parents immigrated and worked multiple jobs to provide opportunities

- Unspoken expectations: Alex should choose career that guarantees middle-class lifestyle

197

Alex's Autonomy-Respect Balance: "I want to make my own choice, but I also want to honor my parents' sacrifices. Maybe there's a way to pursue art that also provides financial security, like graphic design or art therapy."

Social Media Influence Mapping

Social media profoundly affects teenage decision-making in ways that adults often underestimate. These tools help teens recognize and thoughtfully evaluate social media influences.

The Instagram vs. Reality Assessment

Purpose: Help teens distinguish between social media presentations and actual lived experiences.

Process:

1. **Social Media Presentation Analysis**: "What would each of your options look like on social media?"

2. **Daily Reality Analysis**: "What would the actual day-to-day experience of each option be like?"

3. **Highlight Reel vs. Behind the Scenes**: "What are the struggles or challenges of each option that wouldn't show up in social media posts?"

4. **Authenticity Check**: "Which choice feels more about creating good social media content vs. living authentically?"

The Influence Source Mapping

Purpose: Help teens identify and evaluate different sources of social influence on their decisions.

Categories of Influence:

- **Direct Peer Influence**: What friends are explicitly saying

- **Social Media Modeling**: What teens are seeing others do online

- **Influencer/Celebrity Modeling**: What public figures are promoting

- **Family Influence**: Spoken and unspoken family expectations

- **Cultural Influence**: Broader cultural messages about success, happiness, etc.

- **Educational Influence**: What teachers, counselors, or other adults are suggesting

Process:

1. **Map Influence Sources**: Identify which categories are affecting the decision and how.

2. **Influence Evaluation**: For each source, ask:

   o How much weight do I want to give this influence?

   o What values or motivations are behind this influence?

   o How well does this influence align with my personal values and goals?

3. **Integration Planning**: How can you make a decision that thoughtfully considers important influences while staying true to yourself?

The FOMO vs. JOMO Analysis

Purpose: Help teens balance Fear of Missing Out (FOMO) with Joy of Missing Out (JOMO) – the satisfaction of choosing focus over endless options.

Process:

1. **FOMO Identification**: "What are you afraid of missing out on with each choice?"

2. **FOMO Reality Check**: "How realistic are these fears? What evidence do you have that you'll actually miss out on these things?"

3. **JOMO Exploration**: "What would you gain by not choosing certain options? What would you get to focus on more deeply?"

4. **Opportunity Cost Assessment**: "Every choice means saying no to something else. What are you comfortable missing out on?"

Example: Sarah's Activity Overcommitment

Sarah is trying to decide whether to quit one of her many extracurricular activities.

FOMO Analysis:

- Fear of missing out on: Leadership opportunities, college application enhancement, social connections, skill development

- Reality check: "I'm so overwhelmed that I'm not doing any of my activities well, so I'm already missing out on the benefits"

JOMO Analysis:

- Joy of missing out on: Constant stress, rushing between activities, never having downtime

- Focus gains: "If I quit debate team, I could put more energy into student government, which I care about more"

Decision: Sarah realizes that trying to do everything means she's not doing anything well, and that choosing focus over breadth might actually serve her goals better.

Future Self Visualization Tools

Helping teens connect current decisions to their future selves improves long-term thinking and reduces impulsive decision-making.

The 10-Year Future Self Interview

Purpose: Help teens consider long-term implications of current decisions by imagining conversations with their future selves.

Process:

1. **Future Self Development**: "Imagine yourself 10 years from now, living the kind of life you hope to be living."

2. **Future Self Consultation**: "What would 10-years-older you want current you to know about this decision?"

3. **Future Self Priorities**: "What would matter most to your future self about how you make this choice?"

4. **Future Self Gratitude**: "What would your future self thank you for doing? What would they wish you had done differently?"

The Multiple Future Selves Scenario

Purpose: Help teens understand that different choices lead to different versions of their future self, all of which could be positive.

Process:

1. **Future Self A**: "Imagine the future self that results from choosing Option A. What is that person like? What is their life like?"

2. **Future Self B**: "Imagine the future self that results from choosing Option B. What is that person like? What is their life like?"

3. **Future Self Values**: "What values would each future self embody? Which version aligns better with who you want to become?"

4. **Future Self Integration**: "What qualities from both future selves do you want to cultivate regardless of which choice you make?"

The Deathbed Test

Purpose: Help teens consider what will matter most from the perspective of a full life lived.

Adapted from common regret research, made age-appropriate for teens:

Process:

1. **Life Satisfaction Visualization**: "Imagine yourself as an old person, looking back on a life well-lived."

2. **Regret Assessment**: "What would that older, wiser version of yourself regret not trying or not experiencing?"

3. **Pride Assessment**: "What choices would that person be most proud of having made as a teenager?"

4. **Courage Assessment**: "What would that person want to tell current you about taking risks and being brave?"

Note: This exercise should be used thoughtfully and not with teens who are struggling with depression or anxiety about death.

Case Study: Complete Decision-Making Process

Jordan's Post-Graduation Decision:

Jordan, 18, is choosing between taking a gap year to work and travel, attending community college, or going directly to a four-year university. Here's how a complete modern decision-making process might work:

Step 1: Values-Weighted Analysis

Jordan's Core Values: Independence, adventure, financial responsibility, learning, authenticity

Option Scoring:

- Gap year: Independence (9), Adventure (10), Financial responsibility (7), Learning (8), Authenticity (9) = 43

- Community college: Independence (6), Adventure (4), Financial responsibility (9), Learning (8), Authenticity (7) = 34

- Four-year university: Independence (5), Adventure (6), Financial responsibility (3), Learning (9), Authenticity (6) = 29

Step 2: Social Influence Mapping

Peer Influence: Mixed - some friends taking gap years, others going to college *Family Influence*: Parents prefer college but support Jordan's choice *Social Media Influence*: Seeing gap year travel posts looks appealing, college posts look fun but stressful *Cultural Influence*: Messages that college is "normal" path, gap years are risky

Step 3: Future Self Interview

10-Year Future Self Advice: "I'm glad I took time to figure out what I actually wanted before spending money on college. The work and travel experience helped me choose a major I was actually passionate about."

Step 4: FOMO vs. JOMO Analysis

FOMO about gap year: Missing traditional college experience with friends *JOMO about gap year*: Not rushing into expensive education without clear direction, getting real-world experience

Step 5: Integration and Decision

Jordan's Reflection: "The values analysis and future self interview both point toward the gap year. My biggest concern is social - not having the same experiences as friends. But I think I'd regret not taking this chance to travel and figure out what I want more than I'd regret delaying college by a year."

Decision: Gap year with structured plan including work, travel, and college application process for following year.

Teaching Decision-Making Skills for Life

The goal isn't just to help teens make one good decision – it's to help them develop decision-making skills they'll use throughout their lives.

Decision-Making Process Education

Teach the Steps:

1. **Clarify the decision**: What exactly needs to be decided?

2. **Identify values and priorities**: What matters most in this situation?

3. **Generate options**: What are all the possible choices, including creative alternatives?

4. **Gather information**: What do you need to know to decide wisely?

5. **Consider multiple perspectives**: Who else is affected and what are their views?

6. **Evaluate long-term implications**: How will you feel about this choice in the future?

7. **Make the decision**: Choose based on your values and the best information available.

8. **Plan implementation**: How will you follow through on your choice?

9. **Evaluate and adjust**: How is your decision working out, and what adjustments might be needed?

Metacognitive Decision-Making Skills

Self-Awareness Development:

- Recognizing personal decision-making patterns

- Identifying when emotions are helpful vs. problematic in decision-making

- Understanding personal vulnerabilities to certain influences

Process Awareness:

- Knowing when to use different decision-making tools

- Recognizing when you need more information or perspective

- Understanding when decisions can be changed vs. when they're permanent

Decision-Making Confidence Building

Start with Lower-Stakes Decisions: Practice decision-making skills on choices with less permanent consequences.

Celebrate Good Process: Praise thoughtful decision-making processes rather than just outcomes.

Normalize Imperfect Decisions: Help teens understand that most decisions can be adjusted and that perfect choices don't exist.

Build Recovery Skills: Teach teens how to learn from decisions that don't work out as expected.

What Modern Decision-Making Builds Toward

These updated decision-making tools prepare teens for the final step in the change process: translating their decisions into concrete action plans they can actually follow through on.

Understanding what they want to change, how ready they feel, and how to make thoughtful decisions creates the foundation for the practical work of change implementation – setting realistic goals, creating accountability systems, and planning for the inevitable challenges that arise when trying to create lasting change.

Moving Forward with Clarity

The decision-making work you do with teens builds their capacity for thoughtful choice-making throughout their lives. When teens can recognize and evaluate different influences on their decisions, when they can connect choices to their values and future goals, and when they can navigate complex social and family dynamics, they're prepared to create change plans that reflect their authentic priorities and have realistic chances of success.

Chapter 15: My Change Plan

Seventeen-year-old Jasmine has done the work. She's identified her core values (creativity, authenticity, service to others). She's used change rulers to assess her readiness for different changes (importance: 8, confidence: 6 for pursuing art more seriously). She's worked through a modern decision-making process about whether to apply to art schools (decision: yes, along with backup options).

Now she's sitting with her counselor, ready to create an actual plan for making this change happen. But Jasmine has tried to pursue her artistic interests more seriously before, and she's failed. She's set big goals ("I'm going to draw for two hours every day"), made ambitious plans ("I'll build a portfolio in three months"), and then watched herself fall short again and again.

"I know what I want to do," Jasmine says. "But I also know myself. I get excited, I make these huge plans, and then I give up when it gets hard or when other things get in the way. How do I actually make this change stick?"

This is the moment when all the self-awareness, values clarification, and decision-making work gets put to the test. **Creating lasting change isn't about having perfect plans – it's about having realistic plans that account for your actual life, your real strengths and challenges, and the inevitable obstacles that arise when you try to change established patterns.**

The change planning tools in this chapter are designed specifically for teenagers: they account for the realities of teenage life (packed schedules, peer influence, family dynamics), they work with teenage brain development (need for autonomy, social connection, immediate feedback), and they build skills that teens will use throughout their lives.

Understanding Teen Change Challenges

Before creating change plans, it's important to understand why traditional goal-setting approaches often fail with teenagers:

Adolescent Brain Development: The teenage prefrontal cortex, responsible for planning and impulse control, is still developing. This means teens need different kinds of support for following through on goals than adults do (Casey et al., 2019).

Identity Formation Integration: Teen change happens alongside identity development. Changes that feel consistent with emerging identity are more likely to stick than changes that feel imposed or disconnected from sense of self.

Social Context Dependency: Teen behavior is heavily influenced by social context. Change plans that don't account for peer relationships, family dynamics, and school environments often fail regardless of personal motivation.

Perfectionism and All-or-Nothing Thinking: Many teens approach change with unrealistic expectations, leading to discouragement when they don't achieve perfect consistency immediately.

Competing Priorities: Teenagers juggle school, family, friends, work, and extracurricular activities. Change plans that don't account for these competing demands are doomed to fail.

Limited Experience with Change: Unlike adults who have decades of experience with behavior change, many teens are learning change skills for the first time and need extra support for the process.

Teen-Friendly Commitment Tools

Traditional goal-setting formats often feel abstract or overwhelming to teenagers. Teen-friendly tools are concrete, flexible, and designed to work with teenage lifestyles and preferences.

The Change Identity Statement

Purpose: Help teens connect their change goals to their developing sense of identity, making the changes feel personally meaningful rather than externally imposed.

Format: "I am someone who..."

Process:

1. **Current Identity Appreciation**: "What aspects of who you are now do you want to maintain and strengthen?"

2. **Growth Identity Visioning**: "What kind of person do you want to become through this change?"

3. **Identity Statement Creation**: "Complete this sentence: 'I am someone who...'"

4. **Behavior Connection**: "What would someone with this identity do regularly? How would they approach challenges?"

Example: Jasmine's Change Identity

Traditional Goal: "I will draw for 90 minutes every day and complete a portfolio by June

Change Identity Statement: "I am someone who expresses creativity authentically and shares my artistic vision with others."

Behavior Connections:

- Someone with this identity would practice art regularly, even if just for 20 minutes

- They would share their work with trusted friends for feedback

- They would seek out other creative people to learn from

- They would apply to programs that support their artistic growth

- They would see setbacks as part of the creative process, not evidence of failure

The Minimum Viable Change Approach

Purpose: Help teens start with changes so small they're almost impossible to fail at, building momentum and confidence for larger changes.

Concept: Borrowed from startup methodology, this approach focuses on the smallest possible version of a change that still moves teens toward their goals.

Process:

1. **Identify the Big Change**: What's the ultimate change the teen wants to make?

2. **Scale Down Dramatically**: What's the smallest version of this change that would still count as progress?

3. **Make It Ridiculously Easy**: Reduce the change until it feels almost too easy to skip.

4. **Build Consistency First**: Focus on doing the small change consistently rather than doing big changes occasionally.

5. **Gradual Expansion**: Only increase the change after the small version becomes automatic.

Example: Marcus's Exercise Goal

Big Change: "I want to work out for an hour every day" *Minimum Viable Change*: "I will put on workout clothes when I get home from school" *Rationale*: Once he's in workout clothes, Marcus is much more likely to do some kind of physical activity, even if it's just a 10-minute walk

Example: Sofia's Reading Goal

Big Change: "I want to read for pleasure like I used to" *Minimum Viable Change*: "I will read one page of a book before checking my phone in the morning" *Rationale*: One page is achievable every day and creates momentum for longer reading sessions

The Habit Stack Integration

Purpose: Help teens attach new behaviors to existing habits rather than trying to create entirely new routines.

Concept: Based on James Clear's habit stacking, this approach links desired changes to behaviors teens already do consistently.

Format: "After I [existing habit], I will [new behavior]."

Process:

1. **Identify Anchor Habits**: What does the teen do consistently every day without thinking about it?

2. **Match Intensity**: Pair small new habits with established small habits, bigger changes with bigger existing routines.

3. **Logical Connection**: Choose anchor habits that make logical sense with the new behavior.

4. **Environmental Support**: Make sure the environment supports the habit stack.

Example: Alex's Creative Writing Goal

Existing Anchor Habit: "I always check Instagram while eating breakfast" *Habit Stack*: "After I check Instagram at breakfast, I will write three sentences in my journal" *Environmental Support*: Keep journal next to phone so it's visible when reaching for Instagram

Example: Jordan's Academic Organization Goal

Existing Anchor Habit: "I always pack my backpack before bed" *Habit Stack*: "After I pack my backpack, I will write tomorrow's three priorities on a sticky note" *Environmental Support*: Keep sticky notes and pen in the same place as backpack

SMART Goals for Adolescents

Traditional SMART goals (Specific, Measurable, Achievable, Relevant, Time-bound) need adaptation for teenage contexts and developmental needs.

Teen-Adapted SMART Goals: SMARTER

S - Specific and Social: Goals should be specific about what the teen will do, and should account for how the goal affects or involves other people in their lives.

M - Measurable and Meaningful: Goals should be measurable in ways that matter to the teen personally, not just objectively trackable.

A - Achievable and Autonomous: Goals should be realistic given the teen's actual life circumstances and should feel like personal choices rather than external requirements.

R - Relevant and Relationship-Aware: Goals should connect to the teen's values and aspirations and should consider how changes might affect important relationships.

T - Time-bound and Flexible: Goals should have timeframes that create accountability without becoming sources of shame if adjustments are needed.

E - Emotionally Sustainable: Goals should account for emotional realities and not require unsustainable emotional labor.

R - Recovery-Planned: Goals should include explicit plans for how to get back on track after inevitable setbacks.

SMARTER Goal Examples

Traditional SMART Goal: "I will exercise for 45 minutes, 5 days per week, for the next 3 months."

Teen SMARTER Goal: "I will do some form of physical activity that I enjoy for at least 20 minutes, 4 days per week, for the next month. I'll track this in a way that feels motivating to me (photos, journal, app), and I'll tell my best friend about my goal so they can support me. If I miss more than two days in a week, I'll check in with myself about what's getting in the way and adjust my approach if needed."

Analysis:

- *Specific and Social*: Defines activity type and involves friend support

- *Measurable and Meaningful*: Trackable in personally motivating way

- *Achievable and Autonomous*: Realistic frequency, chosen activities

- *Relevant and Relationship-Aware*: Involves friend, accounts for social aspects

- *Time-bound and Flexible*: One month commitment with flexibility for activities

- *Emotionally Sustainable*: Allows for enjoyable activities rather than mandating specific exercises

- *Recovery-Planned*: Explicit plan for handling setbacks

Values-Connected Goal Setting

Purpose: Ensure teen goals connect to their authentic values rather than external expectations.

Process:

1. **Values Foundation**: Start with the teen's identified core values from earlier work.

2. **Goal-Values Connection**: "How does this goal connect to what matters most to you?"

3. **Motivation Source Check**: "Is this goal coming from your own values or from what you think you should want?"

4. **Values Consistency Assessment**: "How will achieving this goal help you become more of the person you want to be?"

Example: Emma's Academic Goal

Core Value: Learning and personal growth *Goal Connection Check*: "I want to improve my grades, but is that because I value learning or because I think I should get good grades?" *Emma's Reflection*: "I realized I was focusing on grades instead of learning. My real goal is to understand and remember what I'm studying, not just get A's." *Revised Goal*: "I will spend 30 minutes after each class reviewing and connecting new information to things I already know, because I value actually understanding what I'm learning."

Accountability Partner Agreements

Teenagers are naturally social creatures, and their changes are more likely to succeed when supported by peer relationships. However, teen accountability partnerships need structure to be helpful rather than sources of pressure or conflict.

Choosing Effective Accountability Partners

Peer Accountability Criteria:

- Someone who shares similar values around growth and change
- Someone who can be encouraging without being pushy
- Someone who's reliable about communication and follow-through
- Someone who won't judge setbacks or struggles
- Someone who has their own change goals (mutual accountability works better than one-way)

Adult Accountability Options:

- Parents (if relationship supports rather than creates pressure)
- Teachers or counselors (if teen feels comfortable with this level of sharing)
- Coaches or mentors
- Therapists or other professionals

Structured Accountability Agreements

Purpose: Create clear agreements about how accountability partners will support each other, preventing miscommunication and resentment.

Agreement Components:

1. **Goals Sharing**: What specific goals is each person working on?

2. **Check-in Schedule**: How often will you check in with each other? (Weekly is usually optimal for teens)

3. **Check-in Format**: Text, call, in-person? What questions will you ask each other?

4. **Support Style**: What kind of support does each person want? Encouragement, problem-solving, gentle reminders, celebration of progress?

5. **Boundary Setting**: What should partners NOT do? Common boundaries include no nagging, no judging setbacks, no sharing goals with others without permission.

6. **Setback Response**: How should partners respond when someone is struggling or has gotten off track?

7. **Confidentiality**: What stays between accountability partners vs. what can be shared with others?

Sample Accountability Partner Agreement

Between Maya and Alex:

Goals: Maya is working on reducing social media use before bed; Alex is working on consistent art practice

Check-in Schedule: Sunday evenings, 20-minute phone call

Check-in Questions:

- How did your change goal go this week?

- What went well?

- What was challenging?

- What do you want to focus on next week?

- How can I support you?

Support Style:

- Maya wants: Encouragement and problem-solving help, no judgment about setbacks

- Alex wants: Celebration of progress and creative collaboration, gentle accountability

Boundaries:

- No daily check-ins (too much pressure)

- No sharing each other's struggles with friends

- No guilt trips about missed goals

Setback Response: Ask "What happened and what would help?" rather than "Why didn't you follow through?"

Family Accountability Dynamics

Purpose: Help teens navigate family support for their changes in ways that support autonomy rather than create pressure.

Family Support Agreement Components:

1. **Information Sharing**: What does the teen want to share with family about their goals? What do they want to keep private?

2. **Support Requests**: What specific support would be helpful from family members?

3. **Boundary Setting**: What kinds of "help" would actually be unhelpful or counterproductive?

4. **Progress Sharing**: How and when will the teen update family on their progress?

5. **Setback Response**: How should family members respond when the teen is struggling with their goals?

Example: Carlos's Study Habits Change

Goal: Develop better homework routines and organization
Information Sharing: Willing to share general goal and weekly progress, not daily details *Support Requests*: Help organizing study space, rides to library when needed, celebration of progress *Boundaries*: No daily questions about homework, no checking up on assignments, no comparing to siblings *Progress Sharing*: Weekly family dinner check-ins about how school week went *Setback Response*: "Is there anything you need help with?" rather than lectures about responsibility

Setback Recovery Planning

One of the biggest differences between teens who successfully create lasting change and those who don't is how they handle inevitable setbacks. Teens need explicit planning for getting back on track after they've gotten off course.

Normalizing Setbacks as Part of Change

Setback Reframing: Help teens understand that setbacks are normal parts of the change process, not evidence of failure or lack of willpower.

Change Process Education: Teach teens that lasting change typically involves:

- Initial motivation and early success
- Inevitable obstacles and setbacks
- Learning and adjustment
- Renewed commitment with better strategies
- Gradual progress with occasional challenges

Perfectionism Prevention: Address all-or-nothing thinking that leads teens to abandon change efforts after minor setbacks.

Traditional Thinking: "I missed three days of my exercise goal, so I've failed and should give up." *Recovery Thinking*: "I missed three days, which tells me something about my approach needs adjustment. What can I learn from this?"

The Setback Analysis Process

Purpose: Help teens learn from setbacks rather than just feeling bad about them.

Setback Analysis Questions:

1. **What Happened?**: Describe the setback factually without judgment

2. **Contributing Factors**: What circumstances contributed to getting off track?

3. **Warning Signs**: What early signs indicated this setback was coming?

4. **Learning Opportunities**: What does this setback teach you about your approach to change?

5. **Strategy Adjustments**: What could you do differently to handle similar situations in the future?

6. **Recovery Plan**: What's the smallest step you can take to get back on track?

Example: Jasmine's Art Practice Setback

What Happened: "I didn't do any art for a week during finals" *Contributing Factors*: "I was stressed about tests, staying up late studying, and my art supplies weren't easily accessible" *Warning*

Signs: "I started skipping art sessions when I felt busy, telling myself I'd make up for it later" *Learning*: "My art practice needs to be flexible during high-stress times, and I need my supplies more accessible" *Strategy Adjustments*: "During stressful weeks, I'll aim for 10-minute sketching instead of longer sessions, and I'll keep a sketchbook in my backpack" *Recovery Plan*: "Tomorrow I'll do a 15-minute drawing to get back into the rhythm"

The Restart Ritual

Purpose: Create positive ways for teens to recommit to their changes after setbacks rather than dwelling on guilt or failure.

Components of Effective Restart Rituals:

1. **Acknowledgment Without Judgment**: "I got off track, and that's okay"

2. **Learning Integration**: "Here's what I learned from this experience"

3. **Strategy Updates**: "Here's what I'm going to do differently going forward"

4. **Fresh Start Declaration**: "I'm starting fresh from this moment"

5. **Immediate Action**: Take one small step toward the goal right away

Example Restart Rituals:

Alex's Writing Restart: After missing several days of creative writing, Alex writes one paragraph about what he learned during his break from writing, then immediately writes one page of new creative content.

Maya's Sleep Routine Restart: After staying up late scrolling for several nights, Maya acknowledges the setback, identifies what triggered it (social media stress), adjusts her approach (phone in different room), and goes to bed 30 minutes early that night.

Building Resilience Through Change Experience

Purpose: Help teens develop confidence in their ability to handle setbacks and continue growing through challenges.

Resilience Building Elements:

Self-Compassion Development: Teaching teens to talk to themselves with the same kindness they'd show a good friend facing similar challenges.

Growth Mindset Reinforcement: Emphasizing that abilities and habits can be developed through effort and learning from setbacks.

Identity Flexibility: Helping teens see themselves as people who are growing and changing rather than people with fixed characteristics.

Support Network Utilization: Encouraging teens to use their support systems during difficult periods rather than struggling alone.

Advanced Change Planning Tools

The Change Environment Design

Purpose: Help teens modify their environments to support their change goals rather than relying solely on willpower.

Environmental Design Process:

1. **Current Environment Assessment**: How does your current environment support or hinder your change goal?

2. **Obstacle Removal**: What environmental obstacles can you eliminate or reduce?

3. **Support Addition**: What environmental supports can you add to make your desired behavior easier?

4. **Temptation Management**: How can you manage environmental temptations without requiring constant willpower?

Example: David's Study Habits Environment

Current Environment Assessment: "My desk is cluttered, my phone is always next to me, and I study in my bedroom where I also relax and sleep" *Obstacle Removal*: "Clear desk daily, study in library or dining room instead of bedroom" *Support Addition*: "Set up organized study supplies, use website blockers during study time, create study playlist" *Temptation Management*: "Phone stays in different room during study sessions, social media apps deleted during exam periods"

The Social Environment Change Plan

Purpose: Help teens navigate how their changes might affect their social relationships and how their social environment can support their goals.

Social Change Planning Elements:

1. **Relationship Impact Assessment**: How might your changes affect different relationships?

2. **Support Person Identification**: Who in your life would support these changes?

3. **Challenge Person Management**: How will you handle relationships with people who might not support your changes?

4. **New Social Connections**: What new social connections might support your change goals?

5. **Social Boundary Setting**: How will you maintain your change goals while staying connected to important relationships?

The Motivation Maintenance Plan

Purpose: Help teens plan for sustaining motivation over time, especially during periods when initial excitement wanes.

Motivation Maintenance Elements:

1. **Values Connection Review**: Regular check-ins about how changes connect to core values

2. **Progress Celebration System**: Planned ways to acknowledge and celebrate progress

3. **Inspiration Renewal**: Regular exposure to inspiring examples of others who embody the changes

4. **Challenge Reframing**: Strategies for viewing obstacles as growth opportunities

5. **Support System Activation**: Plans for reaching out to supporters during low motivation periods

Case Study: Complete Change Plan Development

Jordan's Complete Change Plan:

Jordan, 16, wants to develop better relationships with family members after realizing that conflict and distance don't align with their core value of connection.

Step 1: Change Identity Statement

"I am someone who builds strong, authentic relationships with the people I care about, even when it requires difficult conversations or personal growth."

Step 2: SMARTER Goal Setting

"I will have one meaningful conversation with a family member each week for the next month. 'Meaningful' means talking about something that matters to one of us, not just logistics. I'll track these conversations in my journal and notice how they affect our relationships. If I miss a week, I'll reflect on what got in the way and adjust my approach."

Step 3: Minimum Viable Change

"I will ask one family member 'How was your day?' and really listen to their answer, every day when I get home from school."

Step 4: Accountability Partner Agreement

"My older cousin Maya will check in with me every Sunday about how family conversations went. She'll ask what went well, what was challenging, and what I want to try next week."

Step 5: Environmental Design

"I'll put my phone away during family dinner time, and I'll suggest one family activity each week (like a walk or watching a movie together) to create natural conversation opportunities."

Step 6: Setback Recovery Plan

"If I have a big conflict with family or avoid conversations for several days, I'll:

1. Acknowledge that setbacks are normal in relationship changes

2. Think about what triggered the avoidance or conflict

3. Talk to Maya about what happened

4. Restart with the smallest possible step - just asking someone about their day

5. Adjust my approach based on what I learned"

Step 7: Motivation Maintenance

"I'll remind myself weekly that connection is one of my core values, and I'll notice small improvements in family relationships rather than expecting dramatic changes immediately."

What Change Plans Actually Accomplish

The goal of change planning with teenagers isn't to create perfect plans that eliminate all possibility of failure. The goal is to help teens develop skills for thoughtful action planning, realistic goal-setting, and resilient response to setbacks.

These planning skills serve teens throughout their lives as they face increasingly complex decisions and changes. When teens learn to set goals that align with their values, create support systems that respect their autonomy, and recover gracefully from setbacks, they develop capacities that serve them well into adulthood.

Building Lifelong Change Skills

The change planning process helps teens learn that lasting change is:

- A skill that can be developed rather than a character trait you either have or don't have

- More about systems and environment than about willpower and motivation

- More about progress and learning than about perfection

- More sustainable when it connects to personal values than when it's driven by external expectations

- More successful when it includes social support that respects autonomy

When teens experience success with thoughtful change planning, they develop confidence in their ability to create positive changes throughout their lives. They learn to see themselves as people who can grow, adapt, and create the kinds of lives they want to live.

This foundation of change competence, combined with the relationship skills, communication abilities, and self-awareness developed throughout this workbook, prepares teenagers to navigate the challenges and opportunities of adolescence and beyond with greater resilience, authenticity, and effectiveness.

The Journey Continues

The tools and techniques in this workbook provide starting points for ongoing growth rather than final destinations. As teens continue to develop and mature, they'll revisit values exploration, refine their decision-making skills, and create new change plans that reflect their expanding capabilities and deepening self-knowledge.

The most important outcome isn't any specific change teens make using these tools – it's the development of lifelong skills for thoughtful self-reflection, authentic decision-making, and resilient change implementation that serve them well no matter what challenges or opportunities they encounter.

Appendices

Quick Reference MI Techniques

These techniques can be used in brief moments throughout interactions with teenagers. They don't require formal sessions or extensive training – just a commitment to approaching teens with curiosity rather than judgment.

The OARS Techniques Quick Guide

Open-Ended Questions *Purpose*: Gather information and encourage reflection rather than yes/no responses

Effective Examples:

- "Help me understand your experience with..."
- "What's been going through your mind about..."
- "Tell me more about..."
- "What would need to be different for..."
- "How do you see this situation?"

Avoid: Questions that can be answered with one word, questions that assume problems, leading questions that push toward specific answers

Affirmations *Purpose*: Acknowledge teen strengths, efforts, and positive qualities

Effective Examples:

- "I can see this really matters to you"
- "You're thinking carefully about this decision"

- "It takes courage to share something personal like that"

- "You've shown real resilience in handling this situation"

- "I appreciate your honesty about what's challenging"

Avoid: Generic praise ("good job"), affirmations about things the teen hasn't actually demonstrated, comparing teens to others

Reflections *Purpose*: Demonstrate understanding and help teens hear their own thoughts and feelings

Simple Reflections:

- "You're feeling frustrated about..."

- "It sounds like..."

- "You're saying that..."

- "Part of you wants..."

Complex Reflections:

- "On one hand you value independence, and on the other hand you want your parents' approval"

- "You're torn between wanting to fit in with friends and staying true to your own values"

- "It seems like you're questioning whether the effort is worth it"

Avoid: Reflecting things the teen didn't say, adding your own interpretations, reflecting only negative emotions

Summaries *Purpose*: Help teens organize their thoughts and see patterns in their experiences

Summary Structure:

- "Let me see if I understand what you've shared..."

- "On one hand... on the other hand..."

- "What I'm hearing is that you value... and you're also concerned about..."

- "It sounds like you're trying to balance..."

Quick Engagement Strategies

The 2-Minute Check-In

1. **Notice** something specific about the teen's behavior or demeanor

2. **Ask** an open-ended question about their experience

3. **Listen** without immediately problem-solving

4. **Reflect** what you heard

5. **Affirm** something positive you noticed

Example: "I noticed you seem quieter today. What's going on for you? ... It sounds like you're feeling overwhelmed by everything on your plate. I can see you're really thinking about how to manage it all."

The Values Quick-Connect

1. **Identify** a decision or challenge the teen is facing

2. **Ask** about what matters most to them in this situation

3. **Connect** their concern to their underlying values

4. **Explore** how their values might guide their thinking

Example: "You seem conflicted about this choice. What matters most to you in this situation? ... So fairness is really important to you. How does that value apply to the options you're considering?"

The Scaling Quick-Check

1. **Identify** a change or goal the teen has mentioned

2. **Ask** for a 1-10 rating on importance or confidence

3. **Explore** what makes it that number rather than lower

4. **Ask** what would move the number up

Example: "On a scale from 1-10, how important is improving your grades to you personally? ... What makes it a 7 instead of a 4? ... What would need to happen for it to feel like an 8 or 9?"

Common Mistakes to Avoid

The Advice Trap: Jumping to solutions before understanding the teen's perspective *Instead*: Ask "What ideas do you have about..." or "What's worked for you before in similar situations?"

The Interrogation Pattern: Asking multiple questions in a row without listening to responses *Instead*: Ask one question, listen fully, reflect, then ask a follow-up

The Problem Focus: Concentrating only on what's wrong rather than also exploring strengths and what's working *Instead*: "What's going well for you right now?" or "Tell me about a time you handled something like this successfully"

The Expert Position: Acting like you know what's best for the teen *Instead*: "You know yourself better than anyone else. What feels right to you?"

The Motivation Assumption: Assuming you know what motivates the teen *Instead*: "What would make this change feel worthwhile to you?" or "What do you hope would be different?"

Conversation Starters by Topic

Academic Performance and Motivation

Opening the Conversation:

- "I'm curious about your experience with school this year. What's been going well?"

- "Help me understand what learning feels like for you right now."

- "What subjects or activities at school feel most meaningful to you?"

- "When you think about your academic goals, what comes to mind?"

When Grades Are Concerning:

- "I've noticed your grades in [subject] have changed. What's your experience been like in that class?"

- "Walk me through what homework time looks like for you."

- "What makes it hard to stay motivated with schoolwork?"

- "What would need to be different for school to feel more manageable?"

College and Career Planning:

- "When you imagine yourself after high school, what kind of life do you want to be living?"

- "What draws you to [career/college interest]? What appeals to you about that path?"

- "How do you want to balance your interests with practical considerations like finances?"

- "What concerns do you have about making these big decisions?"

Peer Relationships and Social Concerns

Understanding Social Dynamics:

- "Tell me about your friendships right now. What's going well in your social life?"

- "How do you handle it when there's drama or conflict with friends?"

- "What kind of friend do you want to be? What kind of friends do you want to have?"

- "How do you balance being yourself with fitting in with your peer group?"

Social Media and Digital Relationships:

- "What's your experience like on social media? What do you enjoy about it?"

- "How do you handle social media when it's stressful or overwhelming?"

- "Tell me about how you and your friends communicate online vs. in person."

- "What rules or boundaries do you have for yourself around social media use?"

Peer Pressure and Decision-Making:

- "Tell me about a time when you felt pressure from friends to do something you weren't sure about."

- "How do you handle situations where your friends want you to do something that conflicts with your values?"

- "What helps you make your own decisions when friends have strong opinions?"

- "Who in your life supports you in making choices that feel right for you?"

Family Relationships and Home Life

Family Dynamics Exploration:

- "How would you describe your relationship with your family right now?"

- "What's going well in your family relationships? What feels challenging?"

- "Help me understand how your family communicates about important things."

- "What do you wish your family understood better about you?"

Independence and Autonomy:

- "How do you balance wanting independence with maintaining good relationships with your parents?"

- "What areas of your life do you want more control over? What areas are you comfortable with your parents being involved in?"

- "Tell me about how decisions get made in your family."

- "What would healthy independence look like for you right now?"

Family Conflict Resolution:

- "When there's conflict in your family, how does it usually get resolved?"

- "What communication patterns work well in your family? What patterns create more problems?"

- "How do you handle it when your values or goals seem different from your family's expectations?"

- "What would help your family understand your perspective better?"

Mental Health and Emotional Wellness

General Mental Health Check-Ins:

- "How are you taking care of your mental and emotional health these days?"

- "What does stress look like for you? How do you usually handle it?"

- "Tell me about your energy levels lately. What affects whether you feel energized or drained?"

- "What activities or relationships help you feel most like yourself?"

When You Notice Concerning Changes:

- "I've noticed you seem [specific observation] lately. What's your experience been like?"

- "You mentioned feeling [emotion]. Tell me more about what that's like for you."

- "How long have you been experiencing [specific concern]? What do you think might be contributing to it?"

- "What kind of support would be most helpful for you right now?"

Coping and Resilience:

- "What helps you get through difficult times?"

- "Tell me about a challenging situation you've handled well. What strengths did you use?"

- "How do you usually take care of yourself when you're struggling?"

- "Who in your life provides good support when you need it?"

Risk Behaviors and Safety Concerns

Substance Use Conversations:

- "I'm curious about your experiences with alcohol/substances. What have you observed among your friends?"

- "What's your thinking about [specific substance use]? What factors do you consider?"

- "Help me understand the role that [substance] plays in your social life."

- "What concerns, if any, do you have about your own use or your friends' use?"

Sexual Health and Relationships:

- "How comfortable do you feel talking about relationships and sexuality?"

- "What values guide your thinking about romantic relationships?"

- "What questions do you have about healthy relationships, sexuality, or safety?"

- "How do you handle pressure or expectations around physical intimacy?"

Safety Planning Conversations:

- "Help me understand what safety looks like in your daily life."

- "What situations feel risky or concerning to you?"

- "Who could you reach out to if you ever felt unsafe or needed help?"

- "What would you want adults to know about supporting teen safety?"

Identity and Self-Discovery

Values and Identity Exploration:

- "What matters most to you right now? What are your core values?"

- "How would you describe yourself to someone who didn't know you?"

- "What aspects of yourself do you want to develop further?"

- "What kind of person do you want to become as you grow up?"

Cultural and Social Identity:

- "How do different aspects of your identity (cultural, social, family) influence how you see yourself?"

- "What communities or groups do you feel most connected to?"

- "How do you balance different parts of your identity?"

- "What role does your cultural background play in your daily life and future planning?"

Motivation and Change

Exploring Readiness for Change:

- "What changes, if any, are you thinking about making in your life?"

- "What would need to be different for you to feel like you're living according to your values?"

- "Tell me about something you've changed successfully in the past. How did you do it?"

- "What gets in the way when you want to make changes but struggle to follow through?"

Building on Existing Motivation:

- "What changes are you most motivated to work on right now?"

- "How important is [specific change] to you personally, separate from what others expect?"

- "What would success look like to you with [change goal]?"

- "What resources or support would help you make the changes you want?"

Red Flag Warning Signs

Recognizing when teens need immediate professional intervention rather than motivational support is crucial for their safety and wellbeing.

Immediate Safety Concerns

Suicide Risk Indicators: *Require immediate professional intervention*

- Direct statements about wanting to die, kill themselves, or end their life

- Specific suicide plans or methods discussed

- Previous suicide attempts

- Giving away possessions or making final arrangements

- Sudden improvement in mood after period of severe depression (may indicate decision to attempt suicide)

- Increased risk-taking behavior or reckless actions

- Social withdrawal combined with expressions of hopelessness

- Substance use escalation as coping mechanism

- Access to lethal means (weapons, medications, etc.)

Self-Harm Escalation:
- Increasingly severe or frequent self-injury

- Self-harm in visible places or shared on social media

- Using self-harm to cope with any stress or negative emotion

- Inability to stop self-harm despite wanting to

- Self-harm that results in serious injury requiring medical attention

- Self-harm combined with other risk behaviors

- Expressing that self-harm is their only coping mechanism

Psychotic Symptoms:

- Hearing voices or seeing things others don't

- Paranoid thoughts or beliefs that others are plotting against them

- Severe confusion or disorganization

- Disconnection from reality or inability to distinguish fantasy from reality

- Bizarre or inappropriate behavior that represents significant change from baseline

- Severe mood episodes with psychotic features

Serious Mental Health Concerns

Major Depression Indicators: *Require professional mental health evaluation*

- Persistent sad, empty, or hopeless mood lasting more than two weeks

- Loss of interest in previously enjoyed activities

- Significant changes in appetite or sleep patterns

- Fatigue or loss of energy nearly every day

- Feelings of worthlessness or inappropriate guilt

- Difficulty concentrating or making decisions
- Social isolation from family and friends
- Academic performance decline despite previous capability
- Physical complaints without medical cause
- Preoccupation with death or dying

Severe Anxiety Indicators:

- Panic attacks or severe anxiety that interferes with daily functioning
- School avoidance due to anxiety
- Social isolation due to anxiety about social situations
- Physical symptoms (headaches, stomachaches) with no medical cause
- Perfectionism that causes significant distress
- Obsessive thoughts or compulsive behaviors
- Persistent worry that interferes with sleep, school, or relationships

Trauma Responses:

- Re-experiencing traumatic events through nightmares, flashbacks, or intrusive thoughts
- Avoiding reminders of traumatic experiences
- Negative changes in mood and thinking since traumatic event
- Increased arousal and reactivity (hypervigilance, exaggerated startle response)
- Dissociative episodes or feeling disconnected from self

- Regression in behavior or developmental milestones
- Sudden onset of fear, anxiety, or behavioral changes following a specific event

Behavioral and Social Red Flags

Eating Disorders:

- Significant weight loss or gain in short period
- Obsession with food, weight, or body image
- Avoiding eating with others or making excuses about eating
- Excessive exercise or compensatory behaviors
- Frequent bathroom visits after eating
- Mood changes related to eating or body image
- Social isolation related to food or body concerns
- Medical complications from eating behaviors

Substance Abuse:

- Daily or near-daily substance use
- Using substances to cope with negative emotions
- Continued use despite negative consequences
- Inability to control or stop substance use
- Substance use interfering with school, relationships, or responsibilities
- Lying or being secretive about substance use
- Withdrawal symptoms when not using substances
- Engaging in risky behaviors while under the influence

Family and Environmental Concerns:

- Abuse or neglect by family members or caregivers

- Exposure to domestic violence

- Homelessness or housing instability

- Lack of adult supervision or support

- Involvement with child protective services

- Exposure to community violence

- Exploitation by adults (sexual, financial, or otherwise)

Crisis Response Protocol

When Immediate Safety is Concerned:

1. **Stay with the teen** - Don't leave them alone if they're in immediate danger

2. **Call emergency services** (911) if there's imminent risk of harm

3. **Contact crisis resources** - National Suicide Prevention Lifeline (988), Crisis Text Line (text HOME to 741741)

4. **Remove means of harm** if safely possible

5. **Contact parents/guardians** unless doing so would increase danger

6. **Follow up with professional referrals** for ongoing care

When Professional Assessment is Needed:

1. **Express concern directly** - "I'm worried about you and think it would help to talk to someone trained to support teens with these challenges"

2. **Provide specific resources** - Names, phone numbers, and addresses of local mental health professionals

3. **Offer to help with connection** - "Would it help if I called to make an appointment while you're here?"

4. **Follow up** - Check in about whether professional support was accessed

5. **Maintain ongoing support** - Professional help supplements rather than replaces caring adult relationships

Documentation and Communication:

- Document concerning behaviors and statements objectively

- Communicate with other professionals working with the teen (with appropriate releases)

- Know your organization's policies about confidentiality and reporting requirements

- Maintain boundaries while providing appropriate support

Additional Resources and Referrals

National Crisis Resources

Immediate Crisis Support:

- **National Suicide Prevention Lifeline**: 988 (24/7 crisis support)

- **Crisis Text Line**: Text HOME to 741741 (24/7 text-based crisis support)

- **National Child Abuse Hotline**: 1-800-4-A-CHILD (1-800-422-4453)

- **National Sexual Assault Hotline**: 1-800-656-HOPE (4673)

- **National Domestic Violence Hotline**: 1-800-799-7233

- **Trans Lifeline**: 877-565-8860 (crisis support for transgender individuals)

- **TrevorLifeline**: 1-866-488-7386 (LGBTQ+ youth crisis support)

Online Crisis Resources:

- **Crisis Text Line**: crisistextline.org

- **National Suicide Prevention Lifeline**: suicidepreventionlifeline.org

- **Mental Health America**: mhanational.org/finding-help

- **American Foundation for Suicide Prevention**: afsp.org

Professional Mental Health Resources

Finding Mental Health Professionals:

- **Psychology Today**: psychologytoday.com (searchable database of therapists)

- **American Psychological Association**: apa.org/helpcenter

- **National Association of Social Workers**: helpstartshere.org

- **American Academy of Child and Adolescent Psychiatry**: aacap.org

Specialized Teen Mental Health Programs:

- Many communities have specialized adolescent mental health programs

- Check with local hospitals for adolescent psychiatric services

- Community mental health centers often provide sliding-scale fees

- School districts may provide mental health referral resources

Educational and Academic Support Resources

Learning Support:

- **Learning Disabilities Association**: ldaamerica.org

- **National Center for Learning Disabilities**: ncld.org

- **Understood.org**: understood.org (resources for learning and attention issues)

- Local school district special education resources

College and Career Planning:

- **College Board**: collegeboard.org

- **Khan Academy**: khanacademy.org (free college prep and academic support)

- **Federal Student Aid**: studentaid.gov

- **Career exploration websites**: mynextmove.org, 16personalities.com

- Local community college career counseling services

Family Support Resources

Parent Education and Support:

- **National Federation of Families**: ffcmh.org

- **Active Parenting**: activeparenting.com

- **Love and Logic**: loveandlogic.com

- Local parenting classes through community centers or religious organizations

Family Therapy Resources:

- **American Association for Marriage and Family Therapy**: aamft.org

- **International Centre for Excellence in EFT**: iceeft.com

- Local family service agencies

Substance Use Resources

Teen Substance Use Support:

- **SAMHSA National Helpline**: 1-800-662-4357 (treatment referral service)

- **National Institute on Drug Abuse**: drugabuse.gov/family-checkup

- **Al-Anon/Alateen**: al-anon.org (support for families affected by addiction)

- **Smart Recovery**: smartrecovery.org

Local Resources:

- Community-based substance use treatment programs

- Hospital-based adolescent addiction programs

- Intensive outpatient programs for teens

- Peer support groups for teenagers

LGBTQ+ Support Resources

National Organizations:

- **PFLAG**: pflag.org (support for LGBTQ+ individuals and families)

- **The Trevor Project**: thetrevorproject.org

- **GLAAD**: glaad.org

- **Human Rights Campaign**: hrc.org

Local Resources:

- LGBTQ+ community centers

- Gay-Straight Alliance clubs in schools

- LGBTQ+-affirming religious organizations

- Local pride organizations and events

Technology and Digital Wellness Resources

Screen Time and Digital Wellness:

- **Common Sense Media**: commonsensemedia.org

- **Digital Wellness Institute**: digitalwellnessinstitute.org

- **Center for Humane Technology**: humanetech.com

- Screen time management apps and parental control tools

Cyberbullying and Online Safety:

- **Cyberbullying.org**: cyberbullying.org

- **ConnectSafely**: connectsafely.org

- **National Center for Missing and Exploited Children**: missingkids.org/gethelpnow/cybertipline

Cultural and Community-Specific Resources

Culturally Specific Mental Health Support:

- National Alliance on Mental Illness (NAMI) cultural community pages

- Local cultural community centers and organizations

- Religious organizations providing counseling services

- Culturally competent mental health professionals

Immigration and Documentation Support:

- **United We Dream**: unitedwedream.org

- **National Immigration Law Center**: nilc.org

- Local immigration legal aid organizations

- Culturally competent family service agencies

Financial Resources for Mental Health Support

Low-Cost and Free Mental Health Services:

- Community mental health centers (sliding scale fees)

- University training clinics (reduced-cost therapy with supervised graduate students)

- Religious organizations offering counseling services

- Employee assistance programs through parents' employers

- Medicaid and CHIP coverage for mental health services

Crisis Financial Support:

- Local emergency assistance programs

- United Way organizations

- Salvation Army and other charitable organizations

- Community foundation emergency grant programs

Building Your Local Resource Network

Essential Local Connections:

- Local hospital emergency departments and psychiatric units

- Community mental health centers

- School district counseling and social work staff

- Pediatricians and family medicine doctors who work with adolescents

- Local police and crisis intervention teams

- Child protective services contact information

Professional Development Resources:

- **Motivational Interviewing Network of Trainers (MINT)**: motivationalinterviewing.org

- Local MI training opportunities and consultation groups

- Professional conferences focusing on adolescent development and mental health
- Online continuing education opportunities

Creating Resource Lists for Teens and Families

Customizing Resources for Your Community:

- Research local mental health providers who specialize in adolescents
- Compile transportation options for accessing services
- Identify sliding-scale and insurance-accepted providers
- Create easy-to-access contact information lists
- Update resource lists regularly as services change

Making Resources Accessible:

- Provide resources in multiple languages when possible
- Include websites, phone numbers, and physical addresses
- Consider cultural competence and sensitivity of recommended resources
- Explain what to expect when contacting different types of services
- Include both crisis and non-crisis support options

Using These Resources Effectively

When to Refer

Professional mental health services are appropriate when:

- Safety concerns exist (self-harm, suicide risk, abuse)

- Symptoms interfere with daily functioning for more than two weeks

- Teen or family requests professional support

- Behavioral or emotional changes are severe or persistent

- Multiple areas of functioning are affected (school, relationships, family)

Crisis services are necessary when:

- Immediate safety is at risk

- Teen expresses specific plans for self-harm or suicide

- Psychotic symptoms are present

- Severe substance intoxication creates safety concerns

- Abuse or neglect disclosures require reporting

Building Effective Referral Relationships

Preparation Steps:

- Research local providers and their specialties

- Understand insurance and payment options

- Build relationships with key mental health professionals

- Know the intake processes for different organizations

- Understand typical wait times and crisis availability

Making Successful Referrals:

- Explain the referral process clearly to teens and families

- Provide specific contact information and next steps

- Offer to help with initial phone calls if appropriate

- Follow up to ensure connection was made

- Continue supportive relationship while professional services are accessed

Supporting Teens Through Professional Services

Maintaining Your Role:

- Professional mental health services supplement rather than replace caring adult relationships

- Continue using MI principles in ongoing interactions

- Respect confidentiality between teens and their mental health providers

- Support treatment engagement without taking responsibility for treatment outcomes

- Collaborate with mental health professionals when appropriate releases are signed

The resources and techniques in these appendices are meant to support rather than replace professional training and clinical judgment. They provide starting points for helping teens while recognizing when additional professional support is necessary for safety and optimal outcomes.

Most importantly, these tools are meant to be used within the context of authentic, caring relationships with teenagers. The specific techniques matter less than the underlying respect, curiosity, and faith in teens' capacity for growth that motivates their use.

When adults approach teenagers with genuine interest in their perspectives, respect for their developing autonomy, and commitment to supporting their authentic growth, the specific words and techniques become vehicles for expressing those deeper relational values. That's what makes motivational interviewing with teens effective – not perfect technique execution, but authentic human connection guided by principles that honor adolescent development and potential.

References

Arnett, J. J. (2000). Emerging adulthood: A theory of development from the late teens through the twenties. *American Psychologist, 55*(5), 469–480.

Blakemore, S. J. (2018). *Inventing ourselves: The secret life of the teenage brain*. PublicAffairs.

Blakemore, S. J., & Mills, K. L. (2014). Is adolescence a sensitive period for sociocultural processing? *Annual Review of Psychology, 65*, 187–207.

Brehm, J. W. (1966). *A theory of psychological reactance*. Academic Press.

Carskadon, M. A., Wolfson, A. R., Acebo, C., Tzischinsky, O., & Seifer, R. (2004). Adolescent sleep patterns, circadian timing, and sleepiness at a transitional moment: The start of senior year. *Sleep, 27*(2), 299–310.

Casey, B. J., Galván, A., & Somerville, L. H. (2019). Beyond simple models of adolescence to an integrated circuit-based account: A commentary. *Developmental Cognitive Neuroscience, 17*, 128–130.

Chein, J., Albert, D., O'Brien, L., Uckert, K., & Steinberg, L. (2011). Peers increase adolescent risk taking by enhancing activity in the brain's reward circuitry. *Developmental Science, 14*(2), F1–F10.

Deci, E. L., & Ryan, R. M. (2000). The "what" and "why" of goal pursuits: Human needs and the self-determination of behavior. *Psychological Inquiry, 11*(4), 227–268.

Erikson, E. H. (1968). *Identity: Youth and crisis*. Norton.

Galván, A. (2010). Adolescent development of the reward system. *Frontiers in Human Neuroscience, 4*, 6.

Gunther Moor, B., van Leijenhorst, L., Rombouts, S. A., Crone, E. A., & Van der Molen, M. W. (2012). Do you like me? Neural correlates of social evaluation and developmental trajectories. *Social Neuroscience, 5*(4), 461–482.

Harter, S. (2012). *The construction of the self: Developmental and sociocultural foundations* (2nd ed.). Guilford Press.

LeDoux, J. (2015). *Anxious: Using the brain to understand and treat fear and anxiety.* Penguin Books.

Marcia, J. E. (1980). Identity in adolescence. In J. Adelson (Ed.), *Handbook of adolescent psychology* (pp. 159–187). Wiley.

Rokeach, M. (1973). *The nature of human values.* Free Press.

Small, G., Moody, T. D., Siddarth, P., & Bookheimer, S. Y. (2009). Your brain on Google: Patterns of cerebral activation during internet searching. *American Journal of Geriatric Psychiatry, 17*(2), 116–126.

Steinberg, L. (2013). The influence of neuroscience on US Supreme Court decisions about adolescents' criminal culpability. *Nature Reviews Neuroscience, 14*(7), 513–518.

Steinberg, L., Icenogle, G., Shulman, E. P., Breiner, K., Chein, J., Bacchini, D., ... & Takash, H. M. S. (2018). Around the world, adolescence is a time of heightened sensation seeking and immature self-regulation. *Developmental Science, 21*(2), e12532.

Twenge, J. M., Cooper, A. B., Joiner, T. E., Duffy, M. E., & Binau, S. G. (2019). Age, period, and cohort trends in mood disorder indicators and suicide-related outcomes in a nationally representative dataset, 2005–2017. *Journal of Abnormal Psychology, 128*(3), 185–199.